God. We Still Need You.

God. We Still Need You.

A Year of Pandemic Prayer and Practice From a Hospital Chaplain

Jon Swanson

Contents

Lent

Eastertide

Ordinary Time

The end of the year

Foreword - Curtis Smith

In late fall of 2020, my youngest son left for Air Force basic training. He flew out early one morning, and after a tearful goodbye, an hour later I was at work. At the time, working for Parkview Health, my day started with a taping of *The Daily Dose*, which was a daily video series sent out to all Parkview co-workers. Its purpose was to create connectivity during the pandemic and provide a moment of prayer for the health system in the midst of an enormous crisis.

That morning, I was quite emotional – more than I even realized. The first few people I saw asked me about my son's departure, and as I went to open my mouth to share the experience, words simply wouldn't come out. My mouth would open; my jaw physically worked, but my mouth wouldn't function. About an hour later, I was sitting on *The Daily Dose* set with Jon Swanson, and finally able to form some words, I explained to Jon how surprised I was at my inability to handle the emotion and speak.

Jon responded by asking me a question. "Have you ever had a son leave home in the middle of a global pandemic?", Jon playfully wondered, knowing the answer. I smirked, as I quietly said "no" in a tone that let him know I knew he was asking the question rhetorically. Jon's point was well taken. Circumstances matter, and we don't live our lives in a vacuum.

More than most people I have ever met, Jon understands that reality. He is incredibly intelligent, but it is his emotional intelligence which most impresses me. He always seems to be processing how outside forces are impacting people. More than that, and the thing that most impresses me, is how Jon then turns that understanding into thoughtful prayer and care for other people. Jon leans on God and talks with Him in a meaningful way. I pray daily, and many times I see the way I pray falls into a routine way which can diminish my feeling of connectedness with God. I sense Jon never experiences that feeling, because his prayers are purposeful, thoughtful, unique, and powerful.

I hope as you read this book, you appreciate Jon for the same reasons I do. But more than that, I hope this book touches you and enhances your prayer life. I know that is Jon's hope too.

+++

Curtis Smith is Chief Marketing and Communications Officer for Lasting Change, Inc. During the time of this book, he was Corporate Director of Community Engagement for Parkview Health. Drawing on his years of television experience in Fort Wayne, Curtis was the co-creator and producer of The Daily Dose, a daily video program to encourage Parkview coworkers.

Introduction: The Scribe

"Trauma Team Activate, Level One, 5 minutes, Room 24."

The overhead announcement in the emergency department is simple. It's repeated, in case people missed part of it. Pagers all over the hospital show a similar message: "TRAUMA ACTIVATE (ER) (ROOM E24) LEVEL -1 (ETA 5) MVC ADULT (1) PED (0)." In five minutes, an adult who was in a motor vehicle crash will show up at the hospital, and the injuries are life-threatening.

In response to the page, people start moving toward that room from everywhere in the hospital. X-ray. Trauma surgeon. Respiratory. Phlebotomy. Chaplain. In response to the announcement, the people already in the ED get the room ready for the arrival.

Sitting on a metal stool at the side of the room, already wearing a lead apron, is a nurse. During the next fifteen minutes or three hours, that nurse will be listening and typing and occasionally making phone calls. That nurse will never touch the patient, never touch an X-ray machine or ultrasound, never hang a bag of fluids or squeeze the breathing bag that gives life to the patient.

That nurse will listen and type and occasionally make phone calls.

But make no mistake. The work of that nurse is vital to keeping the patient alive.

That's the scribe.

The scribe is listening for announcements of pressures and pulses and typing them into a record of the activate. The scribe is listening for all the medications, with frequency and amounts, and typing them into the record. The scribe is listening for the specialties and scans needed and making phone calls to find doctors and to schedule CT rooms, and then, typing them into the record.

As the activate event unfolds, the scribe will answer questions: "Which CT room is the patient going to?" "What medication was given with what amount how long ago?" "When did we start compressions?"

The result is a record of the actions that brought stability to the patient while in the emergency room.

Far from being a beginner, the scribe is often the nurse lead at the time of the activate, a nurse with the experience and presence to stay attentive in the middle of chaos. As important as hands-on care is, the complete and accurate **record** of that care can be just as life-saving.

The scribe isn't creating a memoir, isn't writing the biography of the patient, isn't giving interpretation of events. The scribe is creating a record of what was happening at a particular time and place. Others can look at that record and provide the interpretation, the framing, the understanding. Others may be able to say, three weeks later, "That care is what led to this outcome." Or, "In the effort to save the life, these are the long-term effects." Or, "We never would have remembered any of this without a scribe."

+++

For several months in 2020, I was looking for a picture or a story or a metaphor for a Bible project I was working on. I've been reflecting about the Bible book of Ezra for several years, trying to understand how we can make sense of the inventories and royal proclamations and personal testimonies that make up that book.[1] One day, I was listening to Christie Watson and Kate Bowler talking about nurses, particularly in the season of pandemic.[2] Christie is a professor of nursing who put on scrubs and went back into caring for patients.

Christie was talking about the importance of remembering the experiences and traumas that nurses are having. And as she was talking, Christie pointed to the role of scribe.

She talked about the value of journaling at the end of a nursing shift, of regularly capturing the events of the day and the feelings of the moment.

---

1. I started working on the project after my book on Nehemiah. I'm still working on it.
2. "Everything happens: a podcast with Kate Bowler", released 11/17/2020. Christie Watson: Bless the Nurses - Kate Bowler Accessed 2/17/2021.

Part of the value is cathartic, of getting it out. But part of the value is having an in-the-moment record of what the pandemic season was like. The record created by a scribe.

Because we will forget. In the euphoria of a vaccine and the freedom that people will feel, the work of those who lived through the worst will be forgotten.

Tragically, the effects of that work will linger for the rest of the lives of those nurses. And respiratory therapists. And intensivists and patient care techs and EVS workers and child life specialists and radiologists and pharmacy techs. And chaplains.

We will all carry with us the pictures of families on the other end of Zoom calls, watching mom as she is taking her last breaths. We will remember the fastidious, almost paranoid attention to donning and doffing protective gear. We will remember the IV poles in the hallways outside rooms with COVID-19 patients. Or, we will forget those moments and be surprised when we suddenly start crying.

We will all carry with us the tension in our bodies we felt as we read our social media feeds talking about a "made-up" virus as we think about its actual cost on the people we took care of inside the hospital.

+++

As I thought about the connection between the ER scribe and the scribe named Ezra, I realized that this book of prayers I had started is the work of a scribe, of both healthcare worker and religious writer.

Each Sunday since September, 2016, I have stood in front of a congregation and camera in our hospital chapel. I read scripture, I pray, I teach. My wife, Nancy, plays a prelude and a postlude and two hymns. When I say "congregation" I mean 2-3 people who come to the chapel, and people who watch live and by recording every day at 10:30 am and 10:30 pm on a hospital channel.

We follow the three-year cycle of readings in the Revised Common Lectionary, starting with the first Sunday of Advent. The prayer reflects my interaction with God, those texts, and the needs of the people in the hospital. There is often chaos and grief in the mornings before I lead the service, so I started writing out my prayers. I wanted to be able to speak coherently to God and people and often to myself.

In 2020, I published a year of those Sunday prayers, for the year 2018-2019 as *God, We Need You: A Year of Prayer in a Hospital Chapel.*[3]

During 2019-2020, the prayers became different as COVID-19 affected healthcare institutions. People stopped coming to chapel, and then stopped coming to the hospital. There was an awareness that it was just Nancy, God, and me in these conversations in the chapel. However, we kept broadcasting. And because I share these prayers at my blog [4], there were people who were reading them (and praying them with me) every Sunday.

In late March 2020, our hospital system began a new project, a daily internal TV program with a conversation between a host and a number of coworkers. Each episode ended with a prayer from a chaplain. I was part of the process and wrote out the prayers that I then prayed on the The Daily Dose. It made sense to include those prayers in a new collection of prayers.

Hope Swanson Smith, our daughter and my collaborator on this collection, began gathering the chapel prayers and the "Daily Dose" prayers. As we talked, we knew that a collection of prayers in a pandemic year needed context. We realized that we needed to add three more components.

First, the posts I wrote at my blogs [5] were part of my work as a scribe. I was interacting with the hospital, the outside world, God, and a parish of people. Gathering those pieces would help us understand a picture of a community in this year.

Second, documenting the events outside the chapel could provide all of us with context as we reflect on these prayers and essays. After significant conversation, we realized that by highlighting the seasons of

---

3. *God. We Need You: A Year of Prayer in a Hospital Chapel.* Emerald Hope Publishing, 2020. This is part of the series, "Resources on Faith, Sickness, Grief, and Doubt" developed with my friends and colleagues Patrick and Kristen Riecke.

4. 300wordsaday.com

5. 300wordsaday.com and socialmediachaplain.com

the church calendar and then adding this context to the introduction of each season would help us all as we reflect. These are like the notes clipped to the beginning of the documents in Ezra, like the paragraph in a forwarded email that gives an explanation.

Third, because these writings reflect my experience in the chapel, we will all learn by hearing from another chaplain. We turned to a chaplain whose experience started at the beginning of this liturgical, and pandemic, year. Jana started her training on December 8, the third Sunday in Advent.

And so, we have *God. We Still Need You: A Pandemic Year of Prayer and Practice From a Hospital Chaplain.*

+++

If I were to put on my communication scholar hat, I would look for threads running through these prayers and reflections. What was on my heart? What was on my mind?

Like all of us, I am only beginning to think about the implications of all the fear and uncertainty and change for us. I am aware that I could read back through these prayers and reflections and plot them against the graphs we are all sick of seeing. I'm intrigued, for example, that words of confession which appeared in nearly every prayer in the first volume have almost disappeared in this one.

I could also plot them against the people I saw before and after death, the coworkers I watched cry, the leaders who were doing the best they could, the people who were absolutely convinced that what we were seeing every day in the hospital didn't actually exist. Personally, during this year, my mother died, and our daughter and son-in-law lost their first child through miscarriage. Thus, personal and public grief are mixed through these prayers.

But I'm not wearing that hat.

Every time I write these prayers, these conversations with God, I am speaking to God on behalf of people I care about and care for. I'm acknowledging our current status and weakness and struggle and asking for help.

I offer them to you as a way to give voice to the challenges in your own hearts and lives.

About the cover:

On December 2, 2020, I was working my way through my own Advent journal.[6] The assignment for that day was simple: for Christmas, rather than starting with a gift list, start with a hope list. For each person on your gift list, write their name, and list one thing that gives them hope.

Hope, our daughter, was the first person on the list. It may have been because she was 3,000 miles from home at that moment. I sent her an email. "Use tea and wine and coffee as the pigments to create some art."

When she asked if I had anything in mind, I said, "I realized that creativity and art encourage you. And I thought, 'What could she use without having to buy stuff' and realized that painting with the pigments on the ground where you are could be a pretty delightful thing"

Three months later, she came to the house with a small box of paper. She spread the pieces on the counter, triangles, squares, and the distinct air of wine and coffee. On top was the work pictured at the heart of the cover of this book.

As Hope said recently, "Wine and coffee became more familiar to people this year for a variety of reasons." Even as we benefit from the stimulation and relaxation, our souls are stained, colored. As the year went on, we used what we had, like grade-school watercolor trays. And yet, creativity and expression are more than the supplies that go into them. The work and rework and play and patterns are essential to the result.

Some acknowledgements:

For those of us who work in healthcare, 2020 has been a challenge. We have attempted to reconcile the service of our coworkers in difficult and terrifying uncertainty with attitudes of denial and disbelief from those outside the hospital. And so, I have to start by recognizing the coworkers of every role who were in my mind and heart as we worked and prayed this year.

6. *Giving a Year Meaning: A Healing Journal for Advent 2020.*

For Nancy, who watched me go into the hospital every shift, and all the rest of the families who watched their families, I'm grateful. And Nancy walked in every Sunday to play the piano and heard me talk.

For Hope Swanson Smith, who is part of this book as book designer and editor and daughter, I am grateful.

For Patrick Riecke and Lydia Miller, my bosses, who give me the freedom to do the service every Sunday, I'm grateful. And for Susie, Kent, Will, Jana, Dan, Brian, and Dave, who have covered the pager Sunday mornings, I'm grateful. And in particular, for Jana Vastbinder who was willing to bring her story of being formed as a chaplain during this most challenging year, I'm grateful.

For Curtis Smith, who wrote the Foreword and created The Daily Dose and provided a voice of calm in conversations with co-workers for more than ten months, I'm grateful.

For the regular readers and encouragers at 300WordsADay.com, I'm grateful.

To God, who is part of every one of these conversations, I'm forever grateful.

Advent

The first Sunday in Advent was November 27, 2019.

As you likely know, Advent describes a few weeks of preparation before Christmas. In the Church calendar, it's the four Sundays preceding Christmas. In church history, it came to be called "little Lent". It was a season of fasting and reflection and prayer. By starting with this preparation, people would be more ready for Christmastide, the twelve days of Christmas.

What we often don't consider is that Advent is about two arrivals of God. Even as we are anticipating Christmas, which is remembering Christ's first coming, we are anticipating Christ's second coming. This looking-forward element can give hope, reminding us that the story isn't yet done. The Incarnation is essential, but it is not the end of the process of redemption (sorry to sound churchy).

+++

Disaster psychologist Jamie Aten talks about disasters that happen in the world and disasters that happen in the body. In his case, his disaster work started by moving to New Orleans about six weeks before Hurricane Katrina hit. And it continued when he was diagnosed with stage 4 colon cancer. Both are disasters, calling for care.[1] He reminds us to attend to both kinds.

As Advent 2019 began, no one knew about 2019 Novel Coronavirus (COVID-19) and severe acute respiratory syndrome coronavirus 2 (SARS-CoV-2). The first case may have only been 10 days along. A natural disaster was starting.

In our personal life, Advent was preceded with Nancy's broken hip in early November. It was the second broken bone in a year. We were looking to Advent to help us heal. That sense of preparation is reflected

1. https://www.jamieaten.com/walkingdisaster, accessed 3/12/2021.

in an essay in this section: How can we live in an awareness that things will change?

And then Advent was disrupted with the death of my mother following a long slow, descent with Alzheimer's disease. Though we were aware that death was inevitable, we didn't know it was imminent. My sisters and I had already planned to have a simple graveside service at the family cemetery plot. We decided to wait until northern Wisconsin warmed up before having the graveside service. It would turn out to be a long wait.

This would be a typical, mixed-emotion, hopeful Advent.

Preparing as the core of Advent (12/3/2019)

I'm not from the tradition of Advent. I'm from a tradition that looks at the words of Jesus in Matthew (the Gospel reading for the first Sunday of Advent) and says, "We could disappear at any time, so don't be doing things that you wouldn't want Jesus to catch you doing."

There is an element of truth, of course, but it's not a very encouraging way to live. It's a "don't get caught" way of thinking, a "look out!" rather than a look forward way of living.

When Jesus talks about being ready, we could say, "You don't know when he is coming. But you do know THAT he is coming. So be ready. Be prepared. Prepare the way of the Lord."

My hospital life has taught me something about life and change and God coming. Two people can be walking, and one can trip and break a hip. Two people can be in a car, and one can walk away, and one can be critically injured. Or worse.

And in those moments, we all discover something about being ready. We meant to finish those projects on the house. We meant to spend more time together. We meant to finish the conversation, to take care of the healthcare representative paperwork. Some people are ready in all of those ways. Most of us are not.

While the coming of God in all His glory hasn't happened to all of earth, everyone who has lived and died since Jesus said those words has an understanding of being surprised at how quickly we might see God.

So what can we learn about being ready for the coming of Jesus, past, present, and future, this advent season? While we are waiting, how can we be getting ready?

The starting point of Advent, this Sunday called Hope, is the reminder that there IS something to hope for, there is something worth waiting for, and we can prepare by being alert.

The disciples, when Jesus died, were heartbroken. The disciples, when Jesus appeared again, were overcome with fear and then joy. The disciples, when Jesus disappeared and the Holy Spirit came, were determined in their work and invigorated in their expectation of seeing him again. For them, the thought of a future in the full presence of God kept them going.

There was a confidence that came from knowing that they would be together and what that meant.

The more we live in a confidence of God's love for us and God's return for us, the more we can let go of the fear of that coming and work on being ready. Which means living the life that God created us for and calls us to live.

A prayer for the first Sunday of Advent

God.

This is the first Sunday of Advent. Some of us call this Hope Sunday. We read about salvation being closer than ever. And we very much want that to be true.
Because it doesn't always feel that way.

In truth, God, many of us are uncomfortable with expectations. We have expected good things, and bad have happened. We have expected the worst and have sometimes been right. We have expected the best and have seldom been right.

At least about the things that matter to us.
Health. Work. Happiness. Plans. People.

Health doesn't last.
Work doesn't satisfy.
Plans fall through.
People disappoint.
Happiness is temporary.

And God, we don't really want to be negative. We want to trust in you. We want to trust people. We want to know that you will lead and guide and rule with peace.

But things look dark.

Which is why we light candles for Advent. Not because they give much light, but because we need to take tiny steps. Instead of being able to declare with confidence, we whisper in the darkness, "You are our hope. Though it is dark now, we trust that your Kingdom is here and is coming."

In this season, use your past coming to Mary and Joseph and your future coming to reign as king to remind us of your daily promise to be with us always, even to the end.

Through Christ our Lord.

Amen.

+++

Reflecting on Isaiah 2:1-5 and Romans 13:11-14

A prayer for the second Sunday of Advent

God.

I am supposed to have answers and clarity and direction. I am supposed to offer structure and encouragement and order. I am supposed to. And I cannot. Or better, at the moment, in this moment, I have few words, little clarity.

I have, we all have, been through weeks that are overwhelming. We have worked long hours. We have faced separation, death, diagnosis, depression, and hundreds of little things that simply didn't work.

We confess that we turn to comparing struggles, looking at how my week was worse that your week, how my dread is worse than your dread.
We confess that we try to be gracious, ignoring our own struggles because others' struggles seem worse, and thereby do more damage to ourselves.

We acknowledge that as we turn toward comparison, we isolate ourselves from each other and from you. We confess that we are wrapped with layers of past pain and current mistrust and anticipation of a future of more of the same.

What we want to be true is that you, the one who gives us endurance and encouragement, will draw us together.

God of hope, fill us with joy and peace. Help us trust in you. Help us not depend on our own attempts at motivation or inspirational posters or wise sayings. Instead, let us overflow with hope by the power of your Holy Spirit.

Because of what was written in the past about you and your work and your promises, help us to turn our minds and tune our hearts to you. Help us know the words of the law and the prophets and the apostles.

Or better, help us listen to David and Isaiah and Paul and Matthew, people who lived lives, who got angry, who felt fear, who saw death, and who learned to trust in you. In their stories, in your words, we will find encouragement and endurance and hope.

We ask through Christ our Lord.

Amen.

+++

Reflecting on Isaiah 11:1-10 and Romans 15:4-13

In lieu of the third Sunday of Advent, a psalm for the sad.

Several days ago, I sat by the bed of a dying woman, same as I often do as a chaplain. This time it was different. She was my mother.

I am not alone in my loss this year.

Many of us read the passages of words of joy the third Sunday of Advent, the one most often called Joy, and we feel off. We listen to the radio, and we hear songs about "the most wonderful time of the year" and "Joy to the world," and we struggle with the demand to be happy. We struggle with feeling judged if we are not.

People who have suffered loss don't want others to be sad. Many of us have really mixed emotions. But we'd rather not be scolded for being sad.

Some of us turn from the happy Psalms like 146, which was read last Sunday, to Psalm 137.

By the rivers of Babylon we sat and wept
when we remembered Zion.
There on the poplars
we hung our harps,
for there our captors asked us for songs,
our tormentors demanded songs of joy;
they said, "Sing us one of the songs of Zion!"
How can we sing the songs of the Lord
while in a foreign land?

If I forget you, Jerusalem,
may my right hand forget its skill.
May my tongue cling to the roof of my mouth
if I do not remember you,
if I do not consider Jerusalem
my highest joy.

Sometimes the holidays feel like torment. We long and ache for home.

But the presence of Psalm 137 in God's hymnal offers us a little lifeline in our grief, that God will not condemn us for not being happy, that God will not leave us during our season of lament.

A prayer for the fourth Sunday of Advent

God.

We come to you today not wanting to inconvenience you.

Like Ahaz, we do not want to ask you for the wrong amount of anything,
The impossible to reach, the open-handed generosity you offer.

We believe we are polite. We believe we do not deserve much, your humble obedient servants.

But what we call respect or humility is, in all honesty, a lack of trust. A fear of betrayal. A history of watching you not do what we want.

And so we cry out desperately at times but expect the other shoe to drop. We ask everyone we know to pray but are resigned to falling three people or three thousand prayers short.

And we miss the hints that you are generous beyond belief, using a measure we cannot comprehend.

You make plans across ages; we want answers in moments.
You work relationships across generations; we want you to fix our happiness now.

Paul points to prophets and promises and a royal baby, and we see the unlikely girl who should have been ashamed.

We confess that we would have condemned you.
We confess that we often ignore you.
We confess that we seldom trust you in the outcomes and in the process.

We ask you, I ask you, to forgive us, to forgive me.
We ask you, I ask you, to help us trust the signs you give us, to ask for what you offer, to receive what you provide.
We ask you, I ask you, to help us remember you when we forget.

We want to be like Paul and Joseph, starting with misguided urgency, ending with confident calm, resting in the center of your inexplicable peace.

Through Christ our Lord,

Amen.

+++

Reflecting on Isaiah 7:10-16 and Romans 1:1-7

Ardis (12/10/2019)

Children of the heav'nly Father
Safely in His bosom gather;
Nestling bird nor star in heaven
Such a refuge e'er was given. [1]

I've known the song my whole life. I'm guessing that my mother knew the song her whole life, too. It's a Swedish song, written while my grandfather still lived in Sweden.[2] I decided to sing it for my mother the other day. I'm not a singer, of course. And it's possible that I've never sung for my mother. But I don't think she knew any different.

God His own doth tend and nourish;
In His holy courts they flourish;
From all evil things He spares them;
In His mighty arms He bears them.

It's an interesting song to sing, full of emotion from the moments we've sung it before. I was afraid that I wouldn't be able to sing, that I would choke up. Particularly sitting with mom for what turned out to be one of the last two times I was with her. And considering the words. When you are sitting with your memory-gapped, life-ebbing mom singing, "from all evil things he spares them", something feels a little off. Until we think about being carried. That feels a little better.

Neither life nor death shall ever
From the Lord His children sever;
Unto them His grace He showeth,
And their sorrows all He knoweth.

Alzheimer's is an embezzler, stealing what's valuable while leaving the appearance of normalcy. While we watched memory and clear reasoning

---

1. "Children of the Heavenly Father", text: Karolina W. Sandell-Berg, published 1858 Translation: Ernst W. Olson, published 1925. In the public domain.
2. https://wordwisehymns.com/2010/10/03/today-in-1832-lina-sandell-born/

slip away, she denied any change. However, God's love for us doesn't depend on our capacity to remember it.

Praise the Lord in joyful numbers:
Your Protector never slumbers;
At the will of your Defender
Every foeman must surrender.

Mom lived 88 years, 71 of them after she decided that she wanted to follow Jesus. I'm pretty sure that when she opened her eyes wide for the last ten minutes of her life on Monday morning, December 9, she was looking for Jesus. Through cataract-cloudy eyes, with hearing-aid unaided ears, through thoughts long past connecting to memory, she was looking to Jesus, to her never slumbering protector, to her heavenly father.

Though He giveth or He taketh,
God His children ne'er forsaketh;
His the loving purpose solely
To preserve them pure and holy.

I said that I sang for my mom the next to the last time I saw her. I also sang for her Monday morning during her last moments. And I sang for me. Aware that though he giveth or he taketh, God his children never forsakes.

How to start writing again (12/19/2019)

To start writing, you put your fingers on the keys and press down. Or hold a pen or a pencil and start filling the blank space to the right of the point (or to the left, perhaps, depending on the language your mother taught you) with letters.

Ah, but that isn't the real question.

The real question is how do you start writing again when you have been writing for years and you stop and you are now in the space after.

Something happened, a bright searing pain, perhaps, an inconsolable loss, an interminable process with an inevitable ending. There is a then and now, a before and since. And there are no words that are sufficient or adequate or summative or appropriate.

There is no desire to inflict the something that happened on others. And yet, the something that happened is there. It is part of you and thus is part of them, at least as far as you are part of them.

I wrote to a friend. "I feel inarticulate," I said. He said, "What you call inarticulate most people call numb."

I said to Nancy, "I can't speak." She said, "You speak through your fingertips."

I keep swiping, which is, I now know, a fundamentally different motion of the finger and of the heart, than putting your fingers on the keys and pressing down.

When you swipe, you are taking in. The distractions from your story, the combat and the chaos and the chuckles and the callings and the cravings and the calm. But if you (actually, if I) swipe too much, something is swiped from me. From my attention, my reflection, my time, my me.

When you put your fingers on the keys and press down, the flow is, or can be, inside out rather than outside in. Finishing the word, the sentence,

23

the paragraph means that you are finishing the thought. Better, you are finding the thought; you, again I, am finding out what I think and what I feel and what I know and don't know.

And so, it turns out that the way you start writing again is that you put your fingers on the keys and press down.

Christmastide and Epiphany

Christmastide starts on Christmas Day. In 2019, it was a Wednesday. It was the first of the twelve days of Christmas, leading to January 6, the Feast of the Epiphany. Epiphany recognizes the day when the magi arrived at the house where Jesus and his parents were.[1] That meeting marks an intersection of Jesus and the Gentiles, the recognition that the king of the Jews was actually a king for all people.

There were two Sundays after Christmas, and then we started Epiphany, counting the Sundays to Lent. In 2020, Lent began on Wednesday, February 26.

It's hard to know from this side of COVID-19 what we were thinking then. The first case was reported in China on December 30, 2019. For those who paid attention, there was a slowly growing awareness that something was coming. But most of us were living in the normal uncertainty of life. In my prayer for January 12, I acknowledged as much: "We confess that we are poor knowers of the future, confused understanders of the present, and self-protecting historians."

The first case of COVID-19 was reported in Washington State on January 20, 2020.[2]

We traveled to southern Texas to visit friends on February 15-19. The biggest uncertainty on those conversations was about the Mexican-US border policies. The news mentioned the virus, but during this season before Lent, it mattered more to the people who were sick and their families than it did to the rest of us.

The first death in the United States wouldn't come until February 29, the first week of Lent.

---

1. Matthew 2:1-12.
2. https://www.nejm.org/doi/full/10.1056/NEJMoa2001191 accessed 2/12/2021.

A prayer for the first Sunday after Christmas Day

God.

The year is almost done.

We know that years don't really contain events, but they are our way of keeping track of what happens. Some of us are relieved that 2019 is almost done. It's been a year with painful moments and tragic events.

Some of us are relieved that 2020 is almost here. It will let us feel like we have a second or fourteenth chance.

As we think through the year, we are aware of worthy and unworthy,

Of failings and being a failure,
Of successes and being a success,
Of boring moments and being a bore,
Of moments and events that we cannot handle.

We are, we confess, afraid.
We are afraid of success, because what goes well might fall apart.
We are afraid of failure, because everyone will see the real us.
We are afraid of death, of dying broken with you angry at us or ignoring us.

We come to you, Jesus, merciful and faithful high priest,
but we're pretty sure that you aren't glad to see us.

Missing completely the fact that you came to us, glad to see us,
willingly living and suffering and dying and rising to become our merciful and faithful high priest.
You understand our ambiguity about years.
You lived through moments just as painful, events just as tragic, time just as boring as ours.

So help us, Jesus, to live in time, to give up fear, to love more, to care more, to rest more next year than this year, next week than this week, life ahead more than life so far.

Let us rest in your grace and mercy, Jesus.

Amen.

A prayer for the second Sunday after Christmas

God.

It's still the first week of the year. We already feel confused and behind.

We're trying to catch our breath. Some of us because of all the chaos. Some of us because we are actually sick. Our minds, our hearts, and our lungs are feeling clogged.

We hear the words about being chosen.

We confess that sometimes sounds like losing. We're picked to be on the team that gets all the trouble. We're on the team that gets misunderstood. We're on the team that has pastors locked up in China, that has leaders executed in Nigeria, that has people displaced in Central America, that has people sick and ignored here. In our town, in this hospital.

God, we confess that we get caught up in assuming that the condition of our health is a measure of your love.

We confess that we assume you don't like underdogs.
We confess that we aren't working hard enough to make you love us, forgetting that you simply love us.
We confess that we confuse the measure of your love with the meeting of our expectations.

God, we come to you poor and lost and confused and lonely.

Fill us with your wisdom.
Open our eyes to your love.
Mark us with your spirit.
Let us rest in you enough to keep doing your work until we find our final rest with you.

Turn our mourning into gladness.
Give us comfort and joy instead of sorrow.
Help us dance, even as we find it hard to walk.

Through Christ our Lord we ask,

Amen.

+++

Reflecting on Jeremiah 31:7-14 and Ephesians 1:3-14

A prayer for the Sunday of the Baptism of Jesus

God.

We know that you are telling a big story. Across lifetimes, across generations, you see how words to one prophet are true five hundred years later. In a first glimpse. And then are true thousands of years later.

We are aware of our story. Which has frustrations that need to be addressed in the next ten minutes.

You work with millions of people, who have millions of problems, who have millions of worries, who have watched pieces come together in ways that only make sense with your involvement.

We are aware that this week bad stuff may happen, perhaps, though maybe not.
We are aware that bad stuff happened last week at the beginning of the week, that by the end of the week was fine. Or wasn't.

We confess that we are poor knowers of the future, confused understanders of the present, and self-protecting historians.

We confess that we struggle to remember all the pieces of your story that Peter remembered. And even when we do remember the pieces, we struggle to see the connection to us now. To our health, to our feelings, to our relationships, to our faith.

We confess, we are grateful for forgiveness, but we aren't always sure we need it.

We confess, we long for the good news of peace, but we are unsure what you mean by it.

We confess, we feel like bruised reeds and smoldering wicks.

And so we come to you today, asking that you not break us, that you not snuff us out.

We ask that you help us know you, in all of you that we can take, and a little more.

We ask that your forgiveness will free us, your love will overwhelm us, your presence will sustain us. For this week, for this day, for this moment.

Through Christ our Lord,

Amen.

+++

Reflecting on Isaiah 42:1-9 and Acts 10:34-43

A prayer for the second Sunday after the Epiphany

Ah God.

I usually work on Sundays. I'm not working today.[1] That feels like something I should have to confess.

You say to Isaiah, for him and for his people, "You are my servant, Israel, in whom I will display my splendor." And I respond like Isaiah: "But I said, 'I have labored in vain, I have spent my strength for nothing at all.'"

But God, you have made us to rest. To work and to rest. To be faithful in showing up and to be faithful by not showing up at work and by showing up elsewhere. With you. With family. With ourselves.

It's a way that you remind us that you are enough for us before we are enough for you. Your grace and forgiveness are sufficient for us before we are sufficient for you. You are measuring out to us with love and attention and rest while we are worrying about measuring up to you.

God, for me and my family and my people, I ask: *May we, at this moment, know you. May we have the peace that passes understanding, the courage to relinquish control, the rest to let us laugh.*

Through Christ our Lord.

Amen.

+++

Reflecting on Isaiah 49:3-4

---

1. I was in Michigan with family on this day.

A prayer for the third Sunday after the Epiphany

God.

We need you.

Sometimes, when we say that, we mean that we need you to do something. Sometimes, when we say that, we mean that we need you to say something, to fix something, to change everything.

But today, this week, this year, we're not sure what exactly we want you to do, how we want you to fix things.

We are aware of the fear of what could happen with spreading disease.
We are aware of the fear for people feeling the earth shake.
We are aware of the courage of people knowing the threats against their lives because they speak of knowing you.
We are aware of random violence in our city. And when we know it's not random, that doesn't make us feel safer.

So what's clear to us is that in our lack of clarity we simply need you.

You are the one who understands what is going on. You are the one who understands how things turn out. You are the one who understands our fears and our frustration and our anger. You understand from the inside and the outside why people do what they do. And you are with us in our fear to give us your peace that passes understanding, to give us your forgiveness that restores relationship, to give us your your words that are so often stunningly perfect when they come through your word and through your people.

Help us to open our hearts and eyes and minds to your presence.
Help us to move our hands and our feet in obedience and welcome.
Help us be with you as you are with us.

We ask this through Christ our Lord.

Amen.

A prayer for the fourth Sunday after the Epiphany

God.

Some of us feel foolish all the time.

We feel insecure and powerless and overwhelmed.

We're just looking for things to make sense. We're just looking for someone to trust. We're just looking for a sign from you.

And you know we'd do just about anything to get your help. We'd do just about anything to fix the things we've broken, to restore the things we've taken away.

We confess, when we hear that you don't want big sacrifices, it doesn't sound right. When we hear that you don't want demonstrations of our seriousness, you don't want pageantry to prove how much we care, it feels off. And when we read that you want us to walk humbly, to love mercy, to act justly, it feels a little foolish.

That's no way to show we're serious.

You want us to love you by loving each other because you love each other.

That's risky and hard and foolish.

To love our children from diapers to disobedience to adult discussions.
To love the merciful action that doesn't deliver the consequence people deserve.
To love the unpopular act of justice which offers hope to excluded people.
To love with cups of coffee and words of encouragement and rides to the grocery and ignoring our preferences in order to give others opportunities to laugh.

This feels a little foolish.

But you choose weak people and simple ways and small acts to bring your kingdom to earth. You chose Mary and Peter and shepherds and lepers and Nazareth and persecutors and us. You chose us.

Help us to choose you.

Through Christ our Lord,

Amen.

+++
Reflecting on Micah 6:1-8 and 1 Corinthians 1:18-31

A prayer for the fifth Sunday after the Epiphany that was published late.

I laughed a little when I woke up Sunday morning and realized that I hadn't published a prayer for the fifth Sunday after Epiphany. In fact, I hadn't even finished it. I was working on other things. That makes the first line of the prayer I finally wrote for Sunday so important. Because it's true. We aren't perfect.

+++

God.

We come to you today aware that we are not perfect.

We hate to say that out loud, not because we think we are perfect, we know we are not.
But when we say it out loud, we are a little afraid that you or someone else will say, "It's about time you noticed."
And will scold us and mock us and shame us.

And as much as we know they are right,
and are already scolding and mocking and shaming ourselves,
it will still hurt.

And we know that you've said that you love us.
But the truth is, we don't believe it.

Or we are waiting for the rest of the sentence, the one that starts with, "I love you, but…"
We are filling in the rest.

We forget that this is what you say:

"I love you AND I died for you AND I'm with you AND I'm coming for you AND you will get sick and die AND it doesn't mean judgment, it means you are human AND I'm with you."

Paul was right, of course, that your overwhelming love sounds foolish and leaves us speechless.

Help us have glimpses of that love today.

Help us live in the peace it provides.

Through Christ our Lord.

Amen.

+++

Prayer reflects a little of 1 Corinthians 2

A prayer for the sixth Sunday after the Epiphany

God.

I wrote this years ago, for a Friday. But I'm out of town today and aware that this is still true. I still struggle with feeling caught up.

So God, please change the days and hear my heart.

+++

It's the end of the week. But I haven't gotten everything done that I would have liked to get done. I have gotten done things that I probably shouldn't have.

I think that Jesus never felt like this on Friday.

I think that when he got to the end of a week, as he prepared for the Sabbath to start, he thought "I did what I needed to do."

Why could he think that and I don't?

I mean, there were people who weren't healed. In fact, the number of people that he healed on the Sabbath suggests that there were people on Friday who were still sick. And there were disciples who were still confused. And there were people who wanted to see him, people who wanted to hear stories, people who were wanting miracles.

And Jesus still was fine with that.

I know that he talked to you all the time. I know that he talked about doing your will, about doing your work.

I'm guessing that's what I'm supposed to do, too. I'm guessing that if, instead of asking you to help me, I asked to help you, I might look at things differently.

And I try. You know I try. But there are entire hours that I don't think about you.

So what if this morning I ask you to help me help you? What if I decide that today, whatever I get done, will be fine? And what if I decide not to worry every moment that I might make you mad but remember that Jesus wasn't always afraid of making you mad. And what if I thank you for what I have, the opportunities I have.

And what if I am grateful for the weekend rather than dreading what's not done.

Okay?

I mean, amen.

A prayer for Transfiguration Sunday

God.

We would love to be on a mountain, away from all the confusion, and completely present with you.

To see you glowing, to be aware of your power, to be aware that you are aware of us.

That would be awesome.

To have the confidence that Peter had, the confidence that Jesus was full of power. To have the confidence that Peter had, of your words being a bright light shining in a dark place.

We are far more aware of the dark place.

Or, more accurately, of a gray place. Things are foggy in our minds, foggy in our hearts, foggy in our lives.

Rather than bold assurance, we talk to you, sometimes, with grief and questions, with confidence and confusion, with hopes and fears for ourselves and others.

We may not often enough confess that sometimes the fog is from our self-created fatigue, as we stay busy, stay up too late.
We may not often enough confess that sometimes the fog is from our self-broken relationships, our unmaintained connections.
We may not often enough confess that sometimes the fog is from allowing the chaos swirling above our heads to enter into our hearts, to cause us to fret.

We confess.

God, this week we begin the season of Lent, a time not of magic but of choosing to focus on what matters most by letting go of what matters less.

Would you help us, by the power of your Spirit, to think about your glory.
About the glory of your self-sacrificial love.
About the glory of your holy motives and pure plans.
About the glory of your us-welcoming, us-washing, us-transforming, us-lifting love.

And, if it please you, could we have a little of that glory linger on our faces as we turn back to our daily lives?

May it be so.

Amen.

+++

Reflecting on Exodus 24:12-18 and 2 Peter 1:16-21

Longing (1/8/2020)

I think that longing might be the opposite of worrying. Or maybe the opposite of complaining or missing or hoping. I'm not sure.

I came across the word as I was reading *Liturgy of the Ordinary* the other day.[1] It stuck in my brain.

I'm well acquainted with grief, both my own and, as a chaplain, that of others. In grief (which is our response to loss), there are layers of feelings. Among them is the sense that this isn't right. Not in the sense of "I've been done wrong to", though that is often part of grief. But more in the sense of "I know that there is disorder because of selfishness and rebellion and evil, but that's not how things were intended to be when God started things." Said more simply, "this is how things are, but not how things are meant to be."

When we have that sense of disorder, "longing" is a way of describing our desire for a recovery of how things were meant to be.

Paul talks about the pain of life, full of persecution and frustration and conflict and resistance. Much of this pain isn't punishment, as some of us assume. It is what life includes. Then Paul writes,

Meanwhile we groan, longing to be clothed instead with our heavenly dwelling, because when we are clothed, we will not be found naked. For while we are in this tent, we groan and are burdened, because we do not wish to be unclothed but to be clothed instead with our heavenly dwelling, so that what is mortal may be swallowed up by life.[2]

This is not the end of the story. There is a restoration, a reconciliation. Not now, but sometime. And certainly. And the word he uses to describe our desire for that is "longing."

I think many of us are longing.

---

1. Tish Harrison Warren, *The Liturgy of the Ordinary*. (Downers Grove: IVP), 2016.
2. 2 Corinthians 5:2-4

Practice love: wash your hands (1/9/2020)

When I wrote something awhile back about visiting people in the hospital, I said that the most practical thing you can do to be helpful is to foam your hands on the way into the room and foam them on the way out.

It doesn't sound very spiritual, I suppose, but it shows profound love and respect for the person you are visiting and the rest of the people you will see.

That comes to mind today because the hospital where I work is very full these days, with people who are there for germ reasons (as opposed to accidents or strokes).[1] As a result, patients, family members, and staff are feeling a bit overwhelmed. Everyone is waiting. Everyone is wondering. A bunch of people are hurting. A bunch of people are doing the best they can to help.

So here are my spiritual suggestions for today, ways to practically follow Jesus.

1. Heal people (I mean, of course, let God heal through you. But if God uses you to do this? Awesome.)

2. Sleep.

3. If you have a fever, stay home. It shows respect for your colleagues and the public and your elderly relatives.

4. Wash your hands.

5. Wear a (surgical) mask. It's important to be vulnerable and honest, of course and not use the masks of "happy all the time"; but but it's also important to not be vulnerable to germs.

6. Don't holler at the triage nurse. It's not their fault we are all

1. Editor's note from 2021: It was flu season. We hadn't yet seen a known case of COVID-19 in the US. Over the next few months, the hospital would continue to be full for germ reasons.

here.

7. Carry your own tissues. Use them. And wash your hands.

8. Take the medicines you are given, follow the directions you are given.

9. Offer as much graciousness as you can possibly offer.

10. Let me know if you are coming to my hospital. I'll do my best to stop by.

Up to me (2/6/2020)

I woke up early, aware of chaos out there. The psalmist said "Don't fret."

I woke up tired from two long days, aware of work, aware of the chaos out there. The psalmist said, "Don't fret."

I woke up early, anticipating a very long day of scheduled activities, aware of the chaos out there. The psalmist said, "Don't fret."

I read about people like me, people like you, getting upset and angry at the words and actions of others and each other. The psalmist says, "Cease from anger and forsake wrath; Do not fret; it leads only to evildoing."

People like me, people like you, write about other people changing, other people stopping, other people repenting. The psalmist says, "Delight *yourself* in the Lord . . . Commit *your* way to the Lord . . .Trust also in Him."

The psalmist is not naïve. There is evil. But the psalmist doesn't let us off the hook if we spend all our energy talking about how crazy *they* are: "Do not fret; it leads only to evildoing."

People like me, people like you, as we stare at our screens getting upset, what can we do? The psalmist turns our attention from them to us. "Trust in the Lord and do good; Dwell in the land and cultivate faithfulness."

Be present with God so you can carry God's presence with you.

+++

Read Psalm 37. And read it again. And again.

A blessing for blankets (2/12/2020)

The card says that the blanket has been blessed by a chaplain. The blanket is part of a bereavement program at our hospital, a way to offer support to families and friends who are walking out of the hospital after watching someone they love die.

A blanket, a hand print, a memory of the heartbeat doesn't fix anything. It doesn't do the one thing that deep down we all want, for people to be fixed and not die.

But the process reminds staff to slow down for the family's sake and their own. And it gives a family, if they want it, something to hold onto.

So how does a chaplain bless a blanket? Are there magical powers that can infuse the blanket like lavender essential oils? Am I creating a holy object that, when it touches the person, heals them?

That was happening in Ephesus during Paul's work there. People would take handkerchiefs and aprons that had touched him to people who were sick, and they were cured.

When I touch blankets, I don't expect the same result.

A couple times I've had the opportunity to bless a pile of blankets, made by people who care for people who need care. As I touch each blanket, moving it from one pile to another, I say something like, "God, the next time a Chaplain sees these blankets, a person will be dying. These will be touched by patient techs and nurses, family members and respiratory therapists, and by a person who will not live much longer. God, would you care for each of those people as they offer care, as they wrestle in these moments? Would you give them peace that passes understanding, courage for loving one another? And would you let people know that you love them? In the name of the Father and the Son and the Holy Spirit. Amen."

The blankets aren't more holy. But the situations in which they will be present have been mentioned to God. And that is holy.

A storm (2/19/2020)

I have lots of thoughts, but can find no single thread. Like waves in the water.

You know the feeling. I know you do. Because I'm getting emails from you and from me.

And I don't want to minimize the struggle you are having at this moment with some platitude.

So, a story.[1]

There was a storm so bad that experienced sailors were in fear for their lives. Real storm, real fear. And Jesus, asleep in the boat, was shaken awake by the sailors. He said, "Peace" to the wind and the waves. And they were still.

And the sailors were more afraid of him than they had been of the storms.

That said, they still struggled to believe him, still struggled to trust him, still had questions and uncertainty.

But they didn't turn away from him, and he didn't turn away from them. Because the story that was happening in their lives wasn't about their career or bodily safety. It was about becoming people who walked with him for the rest of their lives and beyond.

I cannot promise that you will get answers today or healing tomorrow or a job next Tuesday. Not even if you pray really hard.

I can say that I'm confident that the wind and the waves actually stopped that day. And that you can talk to him about it. And that he's not currently asleep in the back of the boat.

1. See Mark 4:35-41.

Lent

The season of Lent started on Ash Wednesday, February 26, 2020.

In a typical year, Lent is a season for reflecting. The first reading in this section, written February 25, 2020, gives suggestions of how to approach that reflection. They are helpful suggestions. for a year when we need to create change in our habits. But during the seven weeks of Lent, our habits were changed for us.

In January 2021, I wrote about Lent, looking back at 2020:

I've struggled to stop and write about Lent, to create the journal, to say, "How can I help my friends think about Jesus right now." Which is hilarious, right? I'd think that I would be doing that all the time, that I would be all in with the process of looking for ways to connect what we know about Jesus with what we know about our lives. Our struggles, our challenges, our lack of connection.

But we've spent the last year uncertain about how to connect with Jesus. It felt like a whole year of Lent, of giving up things, people, activities, identity. The press coverage and conversations have been about whose side Jesus is on, about what church means, about why people should or shouldn't stay connected.

I understand that struggle.

I've spent a lot of time shaking my head about ways that Jesus was invoked in conversations about wearing masks and structures and integrity of voting systems. I prayed with people before they died, with families afterward, and then had to listen to people saying things that I don't want to walk back through.

+++

At the beginning of Lent 2020, we were hearing about COVID-19 in other parts of the country. The first reported death, in Washington state, was on February 29. That was also the date of the first reported case in New York City.

The first reported case in Indiana was on March 6.[1] For those of us in healthcare in Indiana, we knew our lives were changing. On March 13, public events in Allen County were cancelled, including concerts that the Fort Wayne Children's Choir and the Philharmonic Chorus had been preparing for.[2] Our family gathered for dinner, not knowing that it would be months before we would all be together again.

Also on March 13, Breonna Taylor was killed in her home by plainclothes officers executing a "no-knock" warrant regarding the activities of her ex-boyfriend. In the chaos of the pandemic, there was little press coverage of the death. The way this case was handled by Louisville police contributed to calls for police reform as the year went on.

By March 22, we had our first death in Allen County, where I work.

On April 2, there was a "night of worship" in the parking lots around our trauma center, where people gathered in their cars and listened to the music of a local radio station. It came from a desire to be together, somehow, and to do something to help. There were many such actions.

By April 12, Easter Sunday, 109,000 people had died worldwide.[3]

---

1. https://www.coronavirus.in.gov/ accessed 2/12/2021.
2. Nancy, my wife, works for the Fort Wayne Children's Choir. Hope, our daughter and the editor of this book, was planning for the Philharmonic Chorus concert as her last concert in Fort Wayne.
3. https://web.archive.org/web/20200413003444/https://www.aljazeera.com/news/2020/04/trump-warned-early-coronavirus-threat-live-updates-200411231342507.html accessed 2/26/2021

How can I grow during the seven weeks of Lent (2/25/2020)

Lent starts tomorrow. You can ignore this season without shame. However, some of you are leading groups who will be reading *Lent for Non-Lent People.*[1] You may have people who ask, "How do I figure out what to give up?" Or you may be wondering yourself.

A couple general ways to think:

- Simply ask yourself, "What helpful, beneficial action do I know would help my relationship with God and others, but I just forget to do?" Then do that during Lent.

- Set aside fifteen minutes. Go to a place where you won't be interrupted by others. Say out loud, "God, is there something that you'd like me to do or not do for a few weeks that would help me hear you better?" and then just listen to what goes through your heart. (Seriously. I know that your mind will race. You will run through all the things that you hope it isn't. But if you ask again, you will have a growing awareness of one or two things that are possible. Pick one. Just pick one.)

Or, you can get specific.

Read the questions below. See what kind of argument starts in your thinking. Ask yourself and God whether that argument tells you something about some growing that needs to happen. And then consider making a change, just for the next seven weeks.

- How often do you ask others for advice before you ask God for advice? How could you add in the God conversation first?

- How often do you turn to food when faced with a difficult conversation? How could you turn to God?

- How often are you getting riled up as you read something on

1. A book I wrote to help people walk through Lent.

Facebook or Twitter or in the newspaper? How could you back away from the turmoil?

- How often each week are you specifically thanking God for specific things in your life? How could you add in gratitude?

- How often do you sit in a chair for fifteen minutes and read something from the Bible and say to God, "Is there anything in this that you would like me to follow up with?"

- How many weeks do you take a day and use it to stop working and simply live with your family and friends?

- Who are you bitter at? How could you learn to forgive other people as a way of working up to releasing that bitterness?

- How often are you giving time or money to God?

Be specific in your next step. For example, "During the next seven weeks, each time I get to Friday evening, I will light a candle and put away my work for 24 hours."

Let me know if this list helps.

A prayer for the first Sunday in Lent

God.

This is the first Sunday in Lent. And some of us are aware, even more than at New Years, of how hesitant we are about our commitments. Hesitant is a nice way to say it.

We thought about committing to something in order to draw closer to you. To giving up something distracting. To choosing something that would help us focus. We started on Wednesday. We're uncertain today.

For some of us, we're blaming our weakness.
For others of us, we're blaming the media for drawing us into arguments.
For still others of us, we're wrestling with whether Lent is even an important thing.

I'm not sure, for sure, that you care about Lent. Which is funny, God, since I wrote a book about Lent. But it's not a season you designated. I'm completely sure, however, that you care deeply about us. Enough that you offer us grace and righteousness through Jesus. And in your deep care for us, you invite us to reject the things that distract us and turn from the things that destroy us. You invite us to cling to you, to desire to be in conversation with you, to follow you. You invite us to live in the commitments of Lent, even if we call them something else.

Like repentance. Like obedience. Like self-denial. Like love for one another.

We acknowledge that we are human. We confess that sometimes we act like we are gods. We desire to know you better.

In this season and always.

Through Christ our Lord.

Amen.

A prayer for the second Sunday in Lent

God.

Abram was called by you and loved by you and blessed by you.

But you say that it wasn't his amazing personality or his wonderful business skills or his faithful worship that were behind the call and love and blessing.
It was you all along.

We forget that, God.
We work hard sometimes, but sometimes we don't work as hard as we think we should. And we lament that our personalities are mostly boring, and our business skills are run of the mill, and our worship is sporadic, at best.
But it is you all along.

You called Abram, not because his personality was wonderful, but because yours is.
You are a remarkable conversation partner: listening well, willing to speak our language, to wear our bodies.
You loved Abram, not because he was so successful in business but because you love us before we love you, while we are still wrecked.
And you bless us, not because we bless you with song and story, but because you are the one who blesses.

Abraham was a wandering Aramean, and you called him and loved him and blessed him. You talked with him and forgave him and showed patience with him.[1]

And that is what you are willing to do with us.

May we give you a chance.

May we rest in your calling and love and blessing.

1. Deuteronomy 26:1-6

Through Christ our Lord,

Amen.

+++
Reflecting on Genesis 12:1-4 and Romans 4:1-5, 13-17

A prayer for the third Sunday in Lent

God.

We are afraid.
We call it nervous. Or having an abundance of caution. Or being concerned for others. And we know that maybe we shouldn't feel this way. But it's what we feel.

We are afraid.
We are afraid of what might happen to us.
We are afraid of what might happen to people we love.
We are afraid of not knowing what to do when everything is unsettled.
We are afraid of the people who are not afraid, who are not cautious, who mock us.
We are afraid.

God, you are the one who said "Fear not" every time you showed up in a fear-inspiring way. You are the one who said "Perfect love drives away fear."

Hearing those as commands isn't helpful.
But hearing those as promises does help.
Especially when we hear your tone of voice, not ours.

God, I ask for all of us that we will hear your quiet voice with more clarity than we hear the shouting all around us.

I ask for all of us that we will know your love in ways so real that fear starts to slip away.
I ask for each of us that you will offer us the peace that passes understanding, as we turn to you instead of our own understanding.
I ask that you will hold your fearful ones close.

Through Christ our Lord,

Amen.

A prayer for the fourth Sunday in Lent

God.

Help.

We are anxiously waiting, worriedly ready.
We are increasingly dreading an illness we don't understand. Someone understands. Everyone understands.

What we would love, sort of, is for you to make it disappear. Though we fear who would get credit, who would take credit. What we would love, sort of, is for someone to know, for sure, something. And describe what they know in ways that command respect, that demand compliance, that invite conformity.

But we do not know who to trust.

We are like Samuel late in his life.
Samuel was afraid of Saul; the village leaders were afraid of Samuel; Samuel was captivated by the most likely.
Without you, Samuel was unable to see the right step, the bright hope, the chosen one.

Until David was in front of him, and you said, "That one."

God, we are afraid of many. We are captivated by obvious.

We are willing to stop when you say "go", to say "of course" when you say, "not yet", to say, "are you sure?", when you say "that one".
We are unwilling to be willing. We are uncertain to be certain. We are untrusting to trust.
But we want to be certain, to be willing, to trust you.

So I ask you today, for us all, to touch our eyes, to anoint our heads, to help us see your light.

Even in the confusion and dread.

Through Christ our Lord.

Amen.

+++

Reflecting on 1 Samuel 16:1-13

A prayer for the fifth Sunday in Lent

God.

We are tired.

Our bodies are tired from the anticipation of what could happen and from the disruption of all our usual patterns.
Our minds are tired from planning and adjusting and adapting, from practicing patience.
Our hearts are weary with stories of sickness and suffering, income loss and food inadequacies.
Our spirits feel brittle, as if we were looking at the dry bones of dreams and plans and promises.

Some of us are working and worrying more than ever. Some of us have more time and less certainty than we could have ever dreamed.

And some of us are grieving with no usual ways for comfort.

We long for a touch from you. Not just some metaphor.
We long for actual touch.
We want to love you with heart and soul and mind and strength.
We want to love our neighbors.
We really do.

But we are weary in every way we can be.

God, I ask for protection of relationships and bodies.

I ask for creativity and compassion.
I ask for healing and health.
I ask for conversations that surprise us with tenderness, that restore us with laughter, that humble us with generosity, that heal us with compassion.
I ask for a willingness to abandon the drive for understanding and for

lessons to teach and to embrace a settled commitment to love now, you and others.

May we find rest for our bodies and minds and hearts and souls in your love, today and always.

Through Christ our Lord,

Amen.

A prayer for Palm Sunday

God.

We are anxious and nervous and a little bit bored.
We are anxious about how to pay our bills, how to save our jobs.
We are nervous about what we might catch, what our family might come down with.
We are bored because most of the things we used to do to fill our time are not possible.

And we are not certain who to trust.

People tell us that we're going to make it. And we know that not all of us will make it. Some of us will die.
People tell us that we're all in this together, and we feel alone.

The numbers and the answers and the directions change every day, offered by people we are told to trust.

People tell us that you are in control, that you have a plan, that we're supposed to just trust you.

And I want to tell them that when you told Jeremiah to tell the Israelites about your "plans to prosper them and not to harm them, plans to give them hope and a future," most of the people who heard that letter were going to be dead before it happened.[1]

And I want to remind all of us who think we have you figured out that on this day, you came in on a colt accompanied by cheers, and by Friday night you were dead, accompanied by jeers.

So God, we come to you this morning, I come to you this morning, not sure what to ask you. We could ask you to fix things, but you care more about people. We could ask you to keep people from dying, but you

---

1. Jeremiah 29:11

didn't keep yourself from dying. We could ask you to save us, and you would. But it wouldn't look like the saving we want.

God, help us understand the saving you offer. Help us know that you are present, God with us. Help us know you, help us trust you, help us love you, help us.

Through Christ our Lord.

Amen.

Refreshing your life vs refreshing your browser (2/27/2020)

It's a familiar psalm, Psalm 23. We've heard it at funerals, in hospital rooms, in difficult times and not so difficult times.

It came to mind as I thought about what a friend said the other day. He was talking about a group of people waiting to learn about the next step in their career. They learned that they wouldn't hear anything for another week. "When they quit refreshing their browsers," he said, "They were able to relax and focus better."

I thought about the difference between refreshing our browser and refreshing. When we are refreshing our browser, we are looking for something to change. And that change will cause us stress of some sort, good or bad. Whether it's getting the results of the ongoing game, getting the placement information, finding the growing (or not growing) number of likes on our latest contribution, reading the next outrage in the political or cultural or community news, the more we click, the less refreshment we will find.

In contrast, the Psalmist suggests that the Lord-shepherd will restore (refresh) our souls by leading us into good places. Our souls will be refreshed by still waters and green pastures and the presence of God.

It's hard to imagine that kind of refreshment. I see pain and grief and death every shift I work as a chaplain, in every conversation I have about the pain people are finding in their lives.

We cannot choose the time of accidents and deaths and illnesses and the ways that other people make decisions that change our lives. We can, however, choose where we turn for refreshment. If we turn to refreshing the browser, we will increasingly find frustration. If we quiet our hearts, if we ask God to help, we can, one way or another, find refreshment for our souls.

The people behind the percentages (3/13/2020)

Note: I wrote this the week that visitor restrictions began in our county and as frustrations with those restrictions also began.

I serve at Parkview Regional Medical Center as a chaplain. In that role, all the percentages become people. For example, when a treatment has a 99% success rate, we are the ones who talk with the family members of the 1%, who went from being a risk of side effects to being a person. And now a person who left behind people who cared.

In the middle of all the debating of what percentage and how many and who's creating what kind of panic, those of us in healthcare will be doing our best to provide care, not for percentages, but for faces. These restrictions from our health system may feel hard. But we're already pretty busy each shift with the regular flow of patients, people like you, people whom you love. And any percentage increase because of illness that could be prevented actually means more faces that we see.

I understand the arguments about other causes of death about which we should care, the thousands of deaths from those. I understand them because I see them, one face at a time. I'd love to stop lots of behaviors which lead people to our intensive care units and eventually to our morgue. So argue away about what we should do.

But, please remember that after all the arguments and accusations are over, there are still faces with eyes closed and faces with tears. And one health system working on restrictions intended to help us and to help you. And a team of chaplains there all the time.

Practical observations from a hospital chaplain (3/13/20)

Life goes on. And so does death. Even without viruses, we have death. Even with them, we have life.

+++

If you don't have a person designated as your health care representative, please designate, on the form that is legally acceptable in your state or locality, the person who you want to represent your decisions when you cannot represent yourself. If you have been together for twenty years but haven't gotten around to marriage, or are "like family" but aren't, and you want that person to represent you, put it in writing.

Otherwise, as I see regularly, someone who doesn't know you, or perhaps doesn't like you, may have the legal standing to represent you.

+++

There are resources for congregations at coronavirusandthechurch.com.

+++

Grief is the response to loss. And because of cancellations, there is a lot of loss. If you are my age and you remember that one time your brass ensemble won a blue ribbon at a music competition, and it was a highlight of your music career as a tuba player, consider what it means to prepare for that and then not have the opportunity. When competitions and concerts are cancelled, first dates are changed, celebrations of the family member who loved going to the concert are missed. The geographic and group-bound moments you remember as transformational may not be happening for people you care about. So care for them. The loss is real. And so is the grief.

+++

Laughing is delightful. It's freeing. It's relaxing. But not when it's actually mocking. And pointing out how ignorant people are is almost always mocking.

+++

At the end of his life, when Paul knew that he was going to be killed, he still said, "The Lord will rescue me from every evil attack and will bring me safely to his heavenly kingdom. To him be glory for ever and ever. Amen."[1]

He wasn't naïve. He'd seen a lot. But he was quietly convinced.

1. 2. Timothy 4:18

This is hard (3/17/20)

Nancy and I were emailing yesterday. Among other things, we were talking about her office going on vacation and my office not. About the challenges facing families of the kids her organization serves. About the challenges facing everyone in and out of my organization.

"This is hard," she wrote.

And she's right.

I used to tell families who lost a loved one, "I'm sorry for your loss." I still do. But I realized that they needed someone to look them in the eyes and in the heart and acknowledge that "this is hard."

I told a wife last week, "it's okay for you to not know what to do next." After 45 years together, she was at a loss. That is hard.

And *this* is hard. This moment when almost all of our habits and patterns and routines are being disrupted. Most of our ways of dealing with stress are disrupted. Most of our ways of finding encouragement are being disrupted. Most of our jobs, most of our outings, most of our friends, most of our thinking.

At a time when many people gave up social media for Lent because they wanted to control their dependence, it seems that it will be the only way to see people.

This is hard.

I'm not suggesting that we *stay* with hard, of course.

We can figure out how to love one another in remarkably practical ways. Like sending notes. Like making phone calls. Like making pie. Like listening for the need behind the need and responding to it. Like offering forgiveness. Like spending time learning about Galatians or the causes of homelessness or baking bread with as few ingredients as possible and then sharing what you learn. Like giving away money to people who are out of money because we aren't going to the places they work.

All of those are ways to help which we can do because of the hard.

But I am convinced that there is value in listening to the concerns of the person across from you and saying, "this is hard."

I can't tell you (3/20/2020)

I can't tell you everything that happens, everything that's happening, everything that I see when I walk into the hospital these days.

What we're doing, what we're trying, what we're feeling.

Because I can't speak for 13,000 people who make up the we. Because I have no official status. Because if I talk about this or that, someone may use my statement as evidence in an anecdotal argument.

+++

"But at Parkview, they are doing this and seeing that result, so everyone should."

"How do you know?"

"Self-described chaplain and untrained medical observer, Jon Swanson, hinted at it in a typically vague blog post."

+++

I can tell you this, however. People are continuing to live and die, worry and wonder, regret and repent.

And in all the articles about how long and how deep, about which industries need to take which steps, about which entities are messing with what, about which apocalyptic scenario is playing out, I can tell you this: no one knows.

A prayer for wisdom and strength (3/28/20)

In March 2020, in the early stages of stay-at-home orders and "shutdowns," Parkview Health staff began what would become a ten-month endeavor. They called this The Daily Dose. It included conversations with staff members, encouragement, and prayers from members of the chaplaincy staff. This is my first prayer.

God.

You ask us to come to you when we need wisdom.
We need wisdom now that goes beyond our training.
You tell us to come to you when we need strength.
We need our strength renewed
so that we can run and not be weary;
so we can walk and not faint.

You ask us to come to you when we are afraid.
We are afraid, a little, for our friends, for our families, for ourselves,
We need our courage renewed and our hearts encouraged and
a peace that comes when we don't expect it.

We ask for all of these today for each part of our team.

For one more hallway cleaning,
For one more procedure,
For one more day at home,
For one more meal preparation,
For one more activate,
For one more blood draw,
For one more tear,
For one more smile,

We ask for courage and strength and peace.

Amen.

Eastertide

Eastertide is the fifty days between Easter Sunday and Pentecost. The first time this season happened, it didn't have a name. Jesus was present with the disciples for forty of the fifty days. And then, he ascended out of their sight, and they waited in Jerusalem for the next thing to happen. The next thing for them was the arrival of the Holy Spirit.

In 2020, Easter was April 12. Pentecost was May 31.

It was, by all accounts, a very difficult Easter for people who follow Jesus, for people used to particular kinds of celebration. Face-to-face gatherings were limited. Church services happened online or outside. Family gatherings happened outside or online or not at all.

In the hospital, we were continuing to watch cases of COVID-19 increase. There are pictures all of us carry in our minds that cannot be shared with cameras. In our neighborhood, on a run, I took a picture of a sidewalk message: "It will be okay." Within a month, a member of that house would be a COVID-19 death. For those of us caring for the health of a community we live in, this connection between work and life is real.

There was another kind of uncertainty growing during Eastertide. In Minneapolis, George Floyd was murdered on May 25, 2020. Protests started around the country. And protests in Fort Wayne began May 29, 2020. A growing attention to unjust violence connected the deaths of Ahmaud Arbury, Breonna Taylor, George Floyd, and many others to situations we see at work and in our city.

On Pentecost Sunday, we were deeply in need of an awareness of the presence of the Holy Spirit.

A prayer for Easter 2020

God.

We're used to Easter mornings that are full of music and breakfast and baskets and celebration. In fact, we have come to believe that Easter isn't really Easter without all of that happiness and noise.

So when we get to an Easter Sunday morning, and we can't get together, it feels like it isn't really Easter, that we aren't really Christians.

Forgetting that in many parts of the world, Easter doesn't mean chocolate and new suits and pageantry. And forgetting that often, the pageantry and chocolate and new suits didn't mean you.

In this time where everything is disrupted, we're thinking about all our habits, about our expectations, about our routines. We can't do what we usually do. And we feel lost.

But, God, I'm pretty sure that you aren't disappointed that we don't have trumpets.
I'm pretty sure that you aren't missing the pageantry and new suits.
I'm guessing that all along, you didn't care about all that as much as we did.

Could you help us sort out how to love you with all our hearts and souls and minds and strength when we can't put it into singing together or sharing a table?
Could you help us accept that you are honored when we whisper "help" with the little breath we can gather, the edges of our attention after being together all the time, the last of our energy after a long shift?
Could you give us the willingness to set our minds and hearts on things that matter to you, and the clarity to know what that means?
Could you, would you, today, give us rest?

I ask on behalf of me and my family and my co-workers and our patients and our community and the communities of each of those who reads these words.

Through You, Christ, our Lord.

Amen.

A prayer for the second Sunday of Easter

God.

You already know this, but I have to say it out loud:

We feel trapped.
We feel trapped by executive orders to stay in place.
We feel trapped by an invisible virus or our fear of it.
We feel trapped by the loud combative opinions, citing opposing facts and models, of the people around us. People we used to trust but are not certain of.
We feel trapped by all the demands for our money and attention and agreement.
We feel trapped by our inability to keep up.

And we are trapped enough, some of us, that we are ready to explode at someone –You, the "other" side, people we care about and care for, ourselves.
God, our hearts are not glad and our tongues do not rejoice and our bodies do not rest secure. If asked, we could, perhaps, write a song of lament, but we could not join David in a song of praise.

So today, God, I ask that you will somehow walk through the locked door of our upper room and show us your hands and side and say, simply and quietly, "peace be with you."

And when our trapped-induced fear and panic subside, I ask you to help us live as if you are our God, and we are known and loved by you.
Give comfort to the broken-hearted, healing to the sick in spirit, courage to the faithful. Release us from our fear, I ask.

Through Christ our Lord.

Amen.

A prayer for the third Sunday of Easter

God.

I think that we're wrong about you, most of us, most of the time.

We talk as if you are judging us with plague and pestilence.
We talk as if the most important thing to you is gathering in buildings.
We talk as if you are most in love with – or least angry at – one nation or one party or one system. We talk as if you want us to be healthy, wealthy, and wise.

We forget that Peter says that following you makes us foreigners here.
We forget that you were here before there were nations, and you will be here after all allegiances are gone.
We forget that you call us to obey you, each of us and together.
We forget that you love us to death and back again, each of us and together.
We forget that you command us and invite us, and you show us how to love us all, each of us and together.
We forget that you forgive, each of us and together.
We forget that we need to be forgiven, each of us and together.

Help us remember all of this, through Christ our Lord.

Amen.

+++

Reflecting on Acts 2:36-41 and 1 Peter 1:17-23

A prayer for the fourth Sunday of Easter

God.

We wonder all the time why things happen.

Mostly, we wonder why bad things happen.

Good things like flowers happen, and we are glad. We seldom wonder what we did to deserve them. We often think we worked to earn them.

But bad things, like pandemics and accidents and heart illness and cancer and job loss, those things we wonder about.
We wonder what we did wrong.
We wonder what you are doing wrong.
We wonder what you might want in order to do what we want.
A barter of good living for good health?
A promise of right living for a right outcome?

Peter says, "Jesus was doing great stuff and died for doing right."
I'll be honest, God, that's not helpful.
But he – you – didn't stay dead.
And is – you are – a shepherd.

Looking for us in order to heal our broken hearts.
Leading us in order to heal our broken bodies.
Bringing us together in order to heal our broken souls.

Good Shepherd, even though we will still have questions until we die, we want to know that you know. We want to have life to the full. We want to be led to green pastures. We want our souls restored.

Though we say we want lots of other things, we're pretty sure we want you.
If you'll have us.
And you say you will.

Not through our work,
but through Christ our Lord,

Amen.

+++
Reflecting on Psalm 23 and 1 Peter 2:19-25

A prayer for the fifth Sunday of Easter and Mother's Day

God.

I confess. I cannot keep up.

It is, I think, the confession of most mothers I know.

In chaos and questions,
in the uncertainty about their own mothers and their own children,
in the uncertainty about everyone else's mothers and children,
in the uncertainty about themselves,
they confess, they cannot keep up and they are afraid because of it.

God, Peter lived in a time of chaos and questions, too. So did Mary and Esther and Ruth and Deborah and Eunice and Lois and Elizabeth and Joanna and Phoebe and Sarah and Miriam and Abigail.

And Peter spoke to them and us and all of your people with words of courage and promise and peace.

I ask God, for my sisters, for mothers and daughters, that in this chaos and questions you will help them believe and own these words:

You are a chosen people, a royal priesthood, a holy nation, God's special possession, that you may declare the praises of him who called you out of darkness into his wonderful light. Once you were not a people, but now you are the people of God; once you had not received mercy, but now you have received mercy.[1]

I ask this with gratitude for them,

Through Christ our Lord.

Amen.

1. 1 Peter 2:2-10

81

A prayer for the sixth Sunday of Easter

God.

It's really hard for some of us to talk to you right now.

It's not that we don't like you.
It's not that we are angry with you.
It's not that we are bored with you.

I think it's more that we are having a hard time concentrating on anything for very long, and we think that in order to talk to you we need to concentrate on you.
With disruptions with work and church and life,
with frustrations with friends and family and culture,
with uncertainty about the present and the future, it's hard to concentrate.
With questions about who we are and what we are supposed to be about, we struggle to quiet ourselves.

When we come to you with that kind of disruption, we think we ought to confess something.
We should confess a lack of focus.
We should confess a lack of faith.
We should confess a lack of confidence in you.
It's hard to confess all that.

Perhaps because those aren't things to confess.
Perhaps you aren't pointing out our questions as sins.
Perhaps you are calling out to our souls with hope.

Help us, God, to continue to do good.
Help us, God, to find courage in caring.
Help us, God, to find calmness in your presence.

Through Christ our Lord.

Amen.

A prayer for the seventh Sunday of Easter

God.

We don't want fiery ordeals. We don't want any ordeals, actually.

We don't want to be anxious, we don't want to be tested, we don't want to have to be alert, we don't want you to be gone.
Because we like to believe that if you knew what was going on, you would fix it.
If you knew what was going on, it wouldn't be going on.

We don't want to admit that you warned us that things wouldn't be easy.
We don't want to admit how much we want to know the dates and the times that you are going to do things.
We don't want to admit that you actually promised us power.
We don't want to admit that you want us to live with that power and that courage and that alertness and that strength.

God, on this day we ask you to give strength to the people called by your name who are dying for that name around the world.

On this day, we ask you to remind us that our suffering isn't punishment, our resistance isn't futile,
the measure of your love isn't our happiness but our blessing,
and the measure of your blessing isn't our happiness but your presence.
On this day, we ask you to remind us of your calling to you.
On this day, we ask for your courage and encouragement,
for your peace and contentment, for your healing and holiness.

We wait, with all those who know you in every part of the world.

Amen.

+++

Reflecting on 1 Peter 4:12-14, 5:6-11

A prayer for the Day of Pentecost

God.

Most of the time that we turn to you and start talking, we know what we want. We're not shy about wanting to you fix things, to solve pain, to bring blessing. We know exactly what you should do.

That first day of Pentecost the Apostles were in a room together, talking with you, honoring you, expecting you. But I don't know whether they knew what they wanted you to do, what they wanted you to fix, the pain they wanted you to solve.

I think they were waiting for you. Ready to go when you said, ready to do what you said, ready for you.

They were aware that you were telling a massive story that they were part of. They were aware that the story was going to be hard before it was easy. But they were missing a piece. They were missing you.

God, I'm not sure we're ready for you.

I keep thinking about Nehemiah right now.
Nehemiah was doing fine, working hard, following you.
And then he heard that the walls of Jerusalem were broken and the gates were burned and no one was getting the work done.
And he wept and fasted and prayed.

Every day for four months he said to you:[1]

"Lord, the God of heaven, the great and awesome God, who keeps his covenant of love with those who love him and keep his commandments, let your ear be attentive and your eyes open to hear the prayer your servant is praying before you day and night for your servants, the people of Israel.

---

1. Nehemiah 1:5-11

I confess the sins we Israelites, including myself and my father's family, have committed against you. We have acted very wickedly toward you. We have not obeyed the commands, decrees and laws you gave your servant Moses."

And then he said,

"Lord, let your ear be attentive to the prayer of this your servant and to the prayer of your servants who delight in revering your name."

It is my prayer, too. All of it.

For this place, for this city, for this world.

We have sinned. For a long time. We confess. We wait for your Spirit.

Amen.

+++

Reflecting on Acts 2:1-21

A prayer of gratitude (4/13/2020)

God.

We are constantly aware of numbers.
How many cases, how many shifts,
What trends, what patterns, what curve.

How many and how much and how often build our anxiety and intensity,
sometimes so much that we cannot put one thought with another.
Sometimes so much that we cannot put one conversation with another,
one breath with another.

We are grateful for our co-workers, God, who understand the numbers.
We are grateful for our leaders who exercise their wisdom and diligence.
We are grateful for our system which has worked hard,
together, for minutes and hours and days and weeks.

And yet we still worry.

So today, God, I ask for peace that makes no sense, the peace that comes
from you.

In the middle of a storm,
the peace that allows us to concentrate on holding on.
In the middle of a chaotic shift,
the peace that allows us to see and help the patient in front of us.
In the middle of loneliness at home,
the peace that allows us to hear and offer encouragement.
In the middle of our fatigue, the peace that allows us to offer hope to the
co-worker next to us, behind the mask.

God, what we read is that the peace that passes understanding will guard
our minds and hearts in Christ.

So we ask that you will guard our minds and hearts, protect us from

uncertainty and anxiety as we do our work.
And thank you that you've been doing that all along.

Through Christ our Lord.

Amen.

We confess we still worry (4/23/20)

God.

We need you.
We need something or someone to anchor us.
We need something or someone to steady us.
We need something or someone to stop changing all the time.
Because everyone and everything is changing all the time.
We are fretting. On account of evil doers.
And we aren't sure who the evil doers are anymore.
Because the people we thought we should trust, those in charge, those who you gave charge to, are fully human.
Are they scheming or are they planning?
Are they serving us or you or themselves?
Are they in love with you or with the idea of love?
Are they we?
We confess that we are timid.
We confess that we respond more to public opinions than to your clear simple invitations.
We confess that we worry more about how things will turn out than we remember your clear simple declarations: "our Savior, Christ Jesus, who has destroyed death and has brought life and immortality to light through the gospel."
We confess that we don't always understand that clarity, and we don't always believe that death has been destroyed, and we don't always see life and light.
And we confess that we really don't understand the Gospel,
Not in its richness and abundance and power.
But, we confess, we really want to.
May we know your forgiveness.
May we know your salvation.
May we know your calling.
May we know your power and love and self-control.
May we know you,
Even in the rubble.

Even in the pain.
Even in the present.
Through Christ our Lord, we ask.
Amen

+++

Reflecting on Psalm 37, Lamentations 1:1-6, and 2 Timothy 1:1-14

Help us (4/29/20)

God.

We work in spaces from Warsaw to Wauseon to Wabash to Warren.
We work on tendons and tinnitus and toilets and COVID-19 tests.
We work with spatulas and stethoscopes and spreadsheets.

But we care about people. Coworkers, patients, communities.

Today, I ask you to help us to trust: ourselves, each other, you.
I ask you to help us be safe: physically, emotionally, spiritually.
I ask you to help us discern real needs and hidden concerns and underlying risks.
I ask you to give us miraculous patience with you, with each other, with ourselves.
I ask you to give us passion for justice, for mercy, for people.

We ask this through Christ our Lord, who works in our spaces and on our problems and with our tools.

Amen.

A prayer before Pentecost (5/29/20)

God.

It feels like we're asking you for something all the time.

For peace, for courage, for wisdom, for hope.

It feels like the same thing all the time.

But what we know as Parkview co-workers is that we say thank you all the time.

Not always because we agree, but always because we want to be thankful for the other person, for their commitment, for their presence.

And so today, we say thank you to you.

Not because we always understand what is going on, but because we want to be thankful for you, for your commitment, for your presence.

And as we celebrate Pentecost this Sunday, the coming of your Spirit for peace, for courage, for wisdom, for hope,

I say for us all, thank you.

Amen.

Ordinary Time

In 2020, Ordinary Time started June 7, the Sunday after Pentecost. It ended on November 22, the feast of the Reign of Christ.

There is nothing fancy about Ordinary Time.

In the church calendar, it's the time that isn't part of remembering the two big pieces of the work of God in Christ: birth (Advent, Christmas, Epiphany) and death (Lent, Eastertide, Pentecost). Even the English name, "Ordinary Time", refers not to the ordinariness of the time, but to the fact that the Sundays are numbered: "ordinal". So it's the time that is about living rather than anticipating and celebrating.

2020 was anything but ordinary time. The constant tension caused by a desire to "get back to normal" highlights that. 2020 was full of time between big events.

We lived our lives from day to day. Some people reconstructed their lives around staying home. Many people talked about having so much time on their hands. People posted pictures about learning to bake bread, about spending time reading and writing and getting to know family.

The truth is, as people wrote about not being with people, about having all of this time on their hands, I thought "that would be lovely." I am an introspective person. I am an introvert. I need the time to reflect. And it feels like I had almost no time for reflection during ordinary time.

For many of my coworkers, this time was filled with fear of taking the virus home with them after a long shift of caring for people who weren't getting visitors. It was a time of working from home and feeling separated from work-friends and the scary stuff happening inside our facilities. It was a time of understanding that there isn't ever a normal.

We always face sickness and death. But there was now more, and it was different. We always face questions about what we do. But now there were arguments about the existence of a virus which we saw and wrestled with and adapted to every day. We always work to provide care for everyone. But now we were wrestling with questions about justice in our communities and in our own lives.

It was a very uncertain season of Ordinary Time.

A prayer for Trinity Sunday

God.
In the beginning.
In the beginning, you.
In the beginning, things were good.
In the beginning you created creatively. You created vibrantly. You created gloriously. You created potential and reality, and it was very good.

God.
We are not in the beginning any more.
Things feel chaotic more than creative.
Things feel failed and flawed and fearful rather than good.

God.
Your people have sinned, my tribe has sinned, I have sinned. We try to put loving each other at the top of our list, and we cannot do it on our own. We try to put loving you on our list, but we cannot do it on our own. Our ways of thinking and of acting are all muddled up right now.

It feels almost like the beginning, now that I think about it. Our days formless and void, our plans impossible, our relationships uncertain.

And in the beginning you, Spirit, were hovering over the waters. You, Jesus, were there as the word, speaking light and land and life. You, God Almighty, were there with loving powerful presence. And you, God in three persons, invite us into your relationship.

God, may this be the beginning.
Through Christ our Lord.

Amen.

+++
Reflecting on Genesis 1

A prayer for the eleventh Sunday in Ordinary Time

God.

We would love to be a holy nation.

Not our political nation, exactly, since we come from many nations, many ethnicities.

But like you asked Israel through Moses from the mountain at the beginning of their freedom.

"If you will listen to me," you said.
"If you will keep my covenant," you said.
"Then you will be a kingdom of priests and a holy nation."

A whole kingdom of people who would intercede for those around them, who would speak your words of invitation, who would offer a story of being loved by you.

A whole nation chosen from all the nations to show that you start with the bottom of the pile, the refugee, the outsider, the shepherd. And you love through them.

We confess that some of us have assumed that your love for us means we can condemn other people.
We confess that some of us have assumed that your blessing for us means we can be a curse for others.
We confess that some of us have assumed that we are not stewards but owners.
We confess that some of us have missed almost everything you have said.

We have not visited the sick and imprisoned, we have not fed the hungry or sheltered the homeless. We have not cared for widows and orphans. We have not loved those you have loved, we have beaten our neighbors or ignored them rather than bandaging them up and taking them to an inn and arranging for their care. We have not offered healing to the lepers but have avoided them. We have not driven out demons.

We have not.
We have not done what you have asked us to do.
We want to start.
We really do.
We think.

By the power of your Spirit, give us power to obey.

Today.

Through Christ our Lord.

Amen.

+++

Reflecting on Exodus 19:2-8 and Matthew 9:35-10:8

A prayer for the twelfth Sunday in Ordinary Time

God.

Why is the story of injustice toward Hagar in the Bible?
That makes it biblical, at least for some people.
That gives an excuse.

Sarah despised Hagar and made her life miserable in every possible way.
Sarah wanted Abraham to banish Hagar and Ishmael.
And, God, you told Abraham to do it.

You also said that you would take care of them.
But still, you gave him permission to send them to the wilderness,
for Abraham to condone Sarah's hatred.

It's a really bad story for Father's Day, God.

Except.

You said you would care for Hagar and Ishmael, and you did. Before he
was born, after they were sent away. You kept your promise to keep him
safe. You said, in essence, "Release him to me." And, I suppose, he was
safer away from Sarah.

God, trusting you is hard.
When we are poor and needy, when the people we love are poor and
needy, trusting you is hard.

We want to fix things.
We want to change things.
We want to solve our problems.
We want to blame Hagar when we caused the problem ourselves.

We don't know what to do.
So we acknowledge that we are poor and needy.
We acknowledge that you are God.

We surrender our efforts to fix things ourselves.
We ask you to help us be less biblical like Abraham and Sarah
and more biblical like Hagar.

Who heard what you said
and saw what you showed
and did what you said.

And help us care about the Hagars we know,
the victims of our disobedience.

Through Christ our Lord,

Amen.

+++

Reflecting on Psalm 86, Genesis 21, and Romans 6.

A prayer for the thirteenth Sunday in Ordinary Time

God.

In conversation with you one day, someone prayed, "I will sing of the lovingkindness of the Lord forever; To all generations I will make known Your faithfulness with my mouth."[1]

That was the request of my mom, too.

Gathered with three generations of her family, standing in the cemetery where five generations are buried, we remembered her yesterday as we buried her ashes.

But at her request, we remembered you.
And at her request, we remembered us.

She wanted a memorial service that was about you and us, about your faithfulness to many generations, about our opportunity to live well, for you, in our own generation.

We know that each generation, each day, has troubles of its own.
This cemetery has influenza, heart attack, cancer, pneumonia, Alzheimer's, and simply wearing out.
And all of the attending grief.

But we are aware, God, that you have been mindful of us in and through each of these lives and each of these deaths.

May your comfort continue, through the presence of your Spirit, through the resurrection of Jesus, through your ever-telling of our stories.

Amen.

1. Psalm 89:1

A prayer for the fourteenth Sunday in Ordinary Time

God.

I think we are all like Paul some days.

What we want to do, we don't do. What we don't want to do, we do.

I know, God, that Paul wasn't talking about fitness goals or writing goals. He wasn't talking about mid-year resolutions.

He was talking about doing good and doing bad.

"I want to be kind to people who disagree, but when she says those things, I just want to scream at her."
"I want to love my brother, but when my spiritual brother does foolish things, I just have to tell everyone what a fool he is. On Facebook."

I know that you love everyone, God, and you call us to love one another, and you tell us that the way people will know we are your followers is by our love, but you can't expect me to keep that up with everything going on right now.

Except you can. And you do.

We confess that we react with words rather that responding with prayer. We confess that we forget that calling people names and questioning their intelligence and doubting their love for you is sin. I am assuming your role, rather than living in my role.

What we want, deep down, is to be like you, Jesus.
What we want, deep down, is to be unlike us, Jesus.

What you want, deep down, is for us to live like you in our bodies with our skills and our experiences and our relationships and our passion.

What you want for us is to live the life you delivered us for.

May we, today, stop wanting to do good and simply follow you.

Because that is good.

Amen.

+++

Reflecting on Romans 7:15-25

A prayer for the fifteenth Sunday in Ordinary Time

God.

Isaiah describes buds and flowers and singing hills and clapping trees, and people walking into the middle of it with joy and peace.

And we think about it for a moment and say, "That would be nice."

We sigh.

And then we turn from the Bible app to the Facebook app, and we are lost in the worry and the comparisons and the expectations and the condemnation.

We take barely a moment to consider the words you speak before we are inundated with other words, other images, other noise.

God, I cannot fix all the problems I see, all the noise I hear.

But I can lay down my phone.
I can ask you to help me hear you, to remember the words you actually say.
I want to be like the soil where your words of the kingdom can grow. Not hardpacked with traffic, not distracted by noise, not self-condemning.

Instead, open and waiting and seeking.

I ask through Christ our Lord,

Amen.

+++

Reflecting on Isaiah 55, Romans 8, and Matthew 13

A prayer for the sixteenth Sunday in Ordinary Time

God.

We are groaning this morning.

Some of us in this place have the deep groans of hurting bodies.

Many of us have the deep groans of hurting minds, as we do not understand.
Many of us have the deep groans of hurting hearts, as we miss those who have died this week.

We could say "passed on" or "gone to you, Jesus" or "received their earthly reward", but from our perspective, God, with hearts wounded and broken, they died.

In Texas and Vancouver and Atlanta and Fort Wayne, people who know you have watched the death of the ones they love and they groan.

God, we know there will be glory, but the sufferings of this present time feel great.
God, we cry out to you today, saying "Father" with the quiet desperation of those who know you know our loss but who still need your presence.
God, we cry out today for those who are feeling a loss deeper than ours, for whom we can do little but speak to you.
God, we ask you to give us an awareness today of the hope that can sustain us, a glimpse of understanding of the redemption of our bodies.

Remind us today that you are Immanuel, with us now in our groaning and delight, with us always for your glory.

Give our friends who grieve, your peace.

Give our friends who grieve, us.

We ask through Christ our Lord.

Amen.

+++

Reflecting on Romans 8

+++

On Friday, Laurie Reese died in Texas, Gerald Ringenberg died in Fort Wayne, J.I. Packer died in Vancouver, John Lewis died in Atlanta. Different circles, different numbers of followers and books. But we can't let that confuse us. Same Jesus, same faithfulness to their callings.

A prayer for the seventeenth Sunday in Ordinary Time

God.

We often tell you what we want.

Sometimes you ask us what we need.

Jesus, you asked a blind man what he wanted.

Lord, you asked Solomon what he wanted you to give him.

But, we confess, we are often afraid to tell you what we want, because we are afraid you will judge us. Or we are afraid that it won't happen, and you will look bad. Or we are sure that you won't do it, and we'll be angry with you.

But the blind man was honest. He simply wanted to see.
And Solomon was honest. He wanted the wisdom to do the work you called him to do.

So God, help us to be honest in what we ask you to do.

You have commanded us to love one another. And we see more of others that makes us less motivated to love them than ever.

Would you give us, your servants, the wisdom to have insight into how to love? Would you give us the patience to wait out the pain?

You have told us through Paul that nothing can separate us from your love.

So, as we face difficulty, would you give us, your servants, the discernment we need to not blame you or fear your wrath? Would you help us see your frustration in the context of your love rather than your love in the context of some divine trap?

Would you help us be as honest with you as you are with us? And help us remember your love.

Amen

+++

Reflecting on 1 Kings 3:5-12

A prayer for the eighteenth Sunday in Ordinary Time

God.

We read that you are gracious and merciful.
We read that you are slow to anger and abounding in steadfast love.
And that doesn't fit, exactly, with what many of us think.

We are used to hearing about getting things right, or you'll be mad.
We are used to telling ourselves that we better be careful and do this or that right.
We are used to expecting so much of ourselves and others that we feel that we are failing always. And they feel that way too, because of us.

Maybe we need to confess.
Not our failure, but our belief that it makes you mad.
Not our failure, but the things we tell ourselves about ourselves.
Not our failure, but the judgment we offer freely to others about theirs.

God, we confess.
Not because you are angry, but because you are gracious and merciful.
Not to make you love us, but because you are abounding in steadfast love.
Because you invite us to lean forward to hear you speak.
Because you invite us to eat without charging us.

Thank you that you love us.
Help us believe that you do.

Through Christ our Lord, who is that love,

Amen.

+++

Reflecting on Psalm 145:8-9 and Isaiah 55:1-5

A prayer for the nineteenth Sunday in Ordinary Time

God.

Most of us feel like we're not doing very well.

Like Elijah, we think that everyone is against us, and everything is going wrong, and you aren't keeping up your part of the bargain.

The part that says "If we do good things, you'll do good to us. And if we do bad things, you'll ignore them because you love us."

At the moment, we're trying to do good things, but it seems like all we have is bad news. And so we talk to you like Elijah talked to you.

"I've been very zealous," we say. "But all those other people, they are not.
They are forgetting you.
They are making bad choices.
They are, they are, they are.
But I am, I am, I am.
And now they are trying to kill me."

You didn't kill him.
You didn't scold him.

You gently corrected his view of the situation.
You gave him the next steps forward.

We need your forgiveness for anger and for the ways that we provoke it. We need your forgiveness for hatred, which has been part of our lives almost as long as there have been humans. And which has been wrong that whole time.
We need your forgiveness for racism of all kinds, but particularly the kind that denies we are each made in your likeness and are loved by you.

People are dying because of anger and hatred and racism.

We ask for your courage and your compassion and your conviction to carry to people in the places we live and work and think.

We need to know you love us still.
We need to know you are in the quiet.
Help us to be quiet enough to meet you there.

Through Christ our Lord.

Amen

+++

Reflecting on 1 Kings 19:9-18

A prayer for the twentieth Sunday in Ordinary Time

God.

We have always struggled to get along with each other.

If "we" means humans. And "always" means since there have been humans. And "struggled" means argued with and betrayed and preferred and killed and judged and mocked and enslaved and trafficked and dominated and envied. And "get along with" means valued and encouraged and loved and seen your creative work.

God, we are awful to each other.
Group to group.
Nation to nation.
Person to person.
We think it's getting worse, some of us, though only you can make that assessment.

But God, we confess that we hurt each other in ways we don't know.
We confess that we hate in ways that surprise us.
We confess that we overlook the ways to love that you invite us to.

After decades to think about it, Joseph greeted the brothers who betrayed and sold him.
He forgave them.
And he forgave you.
He saw your wisdom through his story, your sustaining through his struggles, your provision through his persecution.

God.
We need to learn how to love right now.
We need to understand how we can forgive.
We need to be guided by your wisdom.
We need to be less awful.
We need tiny miracles.

We ask in the name of the one who is love and forgiveness. We ask through you, Jesus,

Amen.

+++
Reflecting on Genesis 45

A prayer for the twenty-first Sunday in Ordinary Time

God.

We think that we have it bad.

And we do have it hard, often, looking at ourselves, looking in the moment. I remind people often that we cannot compare grief.

That said, the world Moses was born into was pretty rough.

The government wanted him dead before he was born. The government wanted everyone like him dead before he was born. And yet, you provided protection for him according to your desire to bring freedom to the captives.

When Paul talks to us, at your direction, about the faith and grace you have given each of us, I wonder whether any of us are rescued from death to be a Moses?

I confess that most often, I'm devoted to getting by.

Most often, I'm devoted more to maintaining my comfort than renewing my mind. And then I wonder why I'm so aware of inconveniences and annoyances.

God, today, as we think about your rescue of Moses to a life of challenge and waiting and wandering, help us think in new ways that will transform us so we can discern your will and work.

Help us to act in new ways that will offer help to those who need to be loved and served and led and shown mercy.

Accept our sacrifice of ourselves, not being worthless, but as people who know they are loved.

Let us be used by you for the good of others and the glory of you.

As hard as that is to say and understand and do.

Through the model of Christ our Lord.

Amen.

+++

Reflecting on Exodus 1 and Romans 12

A prayer for the twenty-second Sunday in Ordinary Time

God.

For the record, we would love to see a bush that burns without being consumed. Although we would have an explanation for it.

We would love to hear you talk to us, to tell us what you want from us, what we are supposed to do. We would love to hear that you know us.

But, of course, we do know what you want us to do.

You want us to be devoted to one another. You want us to bless those who persecute us. You want us to feed our enemy instead of repaying his evil toward us.
You want us to provoke peace instead of provoking people.
You want us to do what would be nearly impossible without your help.

So I ask you today to help us.
In the way that you helped Moses, help us.
In the way that you helped the disciples, help us.

Not by fixing everything, but by helping us love and care and follow you.

Through Christ our Lord,

Amen.

+++

Reflecting on Exodus 3 and Romans 12

A prayer for the twenty-third Sunday in Ordinary Time

God.

We're waiting for something to break.

Like a storm breaks, and there is a deluge.
Like a wave breaks, and there is a crash.
Like news breaks, and we know everything is going to change.

We have had so many things change this year, so many things be cancelled, so many plans fall apart.
We have anxiety about what could break next.
We scan the news, repeat the fears, make judgments based on the smallest details.

We confess that we do not love our neighbor until we find out whether they agree with us.
We confess that we measure people's value by their allegiances.
We confess, those of us called by your name, that we have allowed your name to be identified with hate, with anger, with shallowness, with fearfulness.
We confess, those of us called by your name, that we have pursued our reputation more than yours, we have put party ahead of persons, we have been rude and mean and comfortable.

Forgive us for our anger and help us replace it with patience.
Forgive us for our pride and help us replace it with humble service.
Forgive us for our silence and help us replace it with your words of peace.
Forgive us for our fearfulness and help us replace it with quiet trust that whatever breaks, you are with us always, even to the end of the age.

We ask this through you, Christ, our Lord,

Amen.

A prayer for the twenty-fourth Sunday in Ordinary Time

God.

We want you to tell us what to do. We want it as clear as a contract. If we do *this*, you will do *that*.
If we eat this and abstain from that, you will do what we ask.
If we vote this way or support that one, you will make us great.
If we buy this or say that, you will make us more than those who don't.

We confess.
We confess that we want to control you.
We confess that we want to believe without acting.
We confess that we want to act without believing.
We confess that we judge more than we forgive, that we overlook more than we forgive, that we want to make contracts with our forgiveness. And our love.

God, we confess that we are awful right now, those of us who call ourselves by your name. We are mean and rebellious and self-righteous and rude. At least in our hearts, even if not in our mouths and our hands and our posture.

God, by your power, humble us. By your peace, heal us. By your presence, hold us.
Help us remember your forgiveness, always available, always offered, always needed by the best and the worst of us.
Help us be aware of your compassion.
Help us be aware of you, each and all of us together.

We ask through Christ our Lord.

Amen.

+++
Reflecting on Romans 14:1-12 and Matthew 18:21-35

117

A prayer for the twenty-fifth Sunday in Ordinary Time

God.

It's been a hard week.

I feel like we say that to you a lot, these days.

We used to be able to predict what would happen in a week. Now we are resigned to 2020 Bingo cards of disaster and disruption.

"Didn't see that coming," we say.
"I thought it couldn't get worse, and then it did," we say.

And I'm not sure what to say to help.

I can't even settle down to ask you, it seems, because I might miss out on some new disaster or death or drama.

I confess.
I confess that we are captivated by our falsified memories of how things used to be.
I confess that we are distracted by our falsified understandings of how things are now.
I confess that we are terrified by our falsified anticipations of how things are going to turn out.
I confess that we are unaware of what it means that you are the same yesterday, today, and tomorrow.
I confess that we are more comfortable with the complaints of the Israelites than with the courage of Paul.

God. We still need you.
We need you to remind us that you have forgiven us already.
We need you to remind us that most of us aren't suffering for our faith, we are suffering for our lack of faith.
We need you to remind us that you love us.

We need you to remind us that there us more ahead of us than behind us.
We need you to remind us that trusting you isn't denying that we hurt,
but is bringing our hurt to you.
We need you.

Amen.

A prayer for the twenty-sixth Sunday in Ordinary Time

God.

"Why did you bring us here to die?"

That's what the people of Israel asked Moses.
That's what we ask you all the time.

"We're here because you brought us here, and now we're going to die."

Although usually we mean that things aren't going our way.

You gave us this job, and now the people are aggravating.
Why did you bring me here to die?
You put us together, and now we are falling apart.
Why did you bring us here to die?
You brought us to this town, we thought.
Why did you bring us here to die?
You gave me this dream, this desire, this falling apart future.
Why did you bring us here to die?

Though sometimes, God, it really is about death.
My child won't make it through the night.
Why did you bring us to this death?

It's hard, God.

And it's really hard to hold in one hand both the grief and the knowledge that you, Jesus, came specifically with a humiliating death in mind.

Why did you come here to die?

So we hold them in two hands, our frustration and your own life.

We ask you to help us find the ways to love the ones we don't love with your powerful and willing self-surrender. Not giving in or giving up, but choosing to surrender for a better good than either of us, than any of us, can comprehend.

And we ask this, knowing that it's often harder than we can imagine, and knowing that you have done the unimaginable first.

Setting aside your privilege and power and status for us.

Help us understand enough to follow you.

We ask this through Christ our Lord.

Amen

+++

Reflecting on Exodus 17:1-7 and Philippians 2:1-13

A prayer for the twenty-seventh Sunday in Ordinary Time

God.

I try to be honest, God, when I talk to you.

I'll be honest. I want to try to be honest.

Today, I need to honestly say, we do not understand what is really going on. In just about anything.

Nations, families, our own hearts, we know there is chaos and uncertainty and question.

We confess.

We are so overwhelmed with theories and choices and demands and attacks that we are not sure what to confess. We are aware that we read your commands to one group, and we know we fall short.

We read that Paul followed those commands and knew that he fell short. We take it on ourselves to look at the lives of others and point out where they fall short.
We look at the Instagrammed lives of others and believe that we fall short.
We confess. We are constantly measuring and constantly calibrating our value by those measures.

And we are losing every time.

Whatever our nation, we cry out to you.
Whatever our family, we cry out to you.
Whatever our heart, we cry out to you.

Give us a glimpse, God, of your glory that we may find courage.

Give us a glimpse, Jesus, of you that we may find you.
Give us the freedom to forget what is behind and to lean toward you.

We ask today and each day,
through Christ our Lord.

Amen.

+++

Reflecting on Exodus 20:1-20 and Philippians 3:4-14

A prayer for the twenty-eighth Sunday in Ordinary Time

God.

We wish you would say something.

In the chaos and storming of social media, we wish that you would say "Stop". Like you did standing in a boat in a lake in Galilee two millennia ago.

And in the sudden calmness, we would say, "God."

And we might weep.

We forget that we can do that ourselves. We live in a story of our own allowance. We are, some of us, in a storm of our own creation. And we can whisper, "stop" and set aside our phone.

But we know that we are beset by storms in our own souls, too. And we forget that one way to talk with you is to start with the torrent of our requests, in prayer and petition.

Not just for a job or a car or a healing. But our deepest fears and our most earnest hopes and our most baffling uncertainties and our middle-of-the-night darkness. We can, Paul says, tell you all of that.

And with no promise of fixing it the way we want, you will place your peace on guard duty for our hearts. You will place your peace as a network security for our minds.

God, I do not know how that works. I do not think it's a contract depending on how much we tell you. I think it's an invitation to be with you.

Help us.

Through Christ our Lord,

Amen.

+++

Reflecting on Philippians 4

A prayer for the twenty-ninth Sunday in Ordinary Time

God.

We are anxious.

We are anxious to and anxious about.
We are longing to and longing for.
And we are, a little, dreading.

Then we read about Moses on a mountain with you.

You tell him you care.

And in the middle of the cloud of your presence, hearing the whispers of your voice, with the experience of eighty years of confirmations and affirmations and appearances and miracles, Moses still asks you for three things:
Show me your ways.
Go with us.
Show me your glory.

That could be a sermon, teaching about you. It could be a lecture, fostering a greater sense of obligation.
Instead it's a prayer for today, with a quiet voice, that is a little anxious.
Show us your ways, please?
Go with us, please?
Show me your glory, please?

Through Christ our Lord.

Amen.

+++

Reflecting on Exodus 33:12-23

A prayer for the thirtieth Sunday in Ordinary Time

God.

I think we really need you.

We are, we admit, weary of all the noise and fear and confusion.

We are weary of our friends yelling at our friends.
We are afraid of what will happen if someone thinks we said the wrong thing.
We are confused by all the opinions and ultimatums and statements which claim to be facts.

We read about Moses who lived 12 decades, knowing you, talking with you, facing noise and fear and confusion.
We read about Paul, who walked into a city and spent time talking about you. And being attacked and criticized and driven out of town.

Following you is hard and unpopular work, apparently.

What comes to mind as we talk, God, is that Moses and Paul spent their time calling the people who know you to obey you rather than trying to change Egypt or Rome.
They spoke of relationship with you, of pouring their lives into conversing with and caring for people.

God, if we quietly, persistently, love our friends, is that what you want?
If we courageously, persistently, speak of your love, is that what you want?
If we consistently, persistently, look into your face and into the faces of our friends rather than trying to respond to and repeat every rumor and opinion and theory, is that what you want?
If we shared our lives like a nursing mother, rather than sharing our opinions like a parrot, is that what you want?

Since that is what you did, Jesus, perhaps it's what you want from us, too.

Give us that awareness of your ways, Jesus,

We ask through your name,

Amen.

+++

Reflecting on Deuteronomy 34:1-12 and 1 Thessalonians 2:1-8

A prayer for the thirty-first Sunday in Ordinary Time

God.

We miss them.

We know, of course, that to be absent from the body is to be present with you.

That's all very well for them, and for you, but we miss our loved ones.

And on this All Saints Day when we have said goodbye to more loved ones that usual, our hearts are unusually sad.

Decades ago, a poet prayed with deep honesty about the tension we feel:

O blest communion, fellowship divine,
we feebly struggle, they in glory shine;
yet all are one in thee, for all are thine.[1]

I ask that you will give us comfort today in the memories we have of those we no longer can see. Help us know the immensity of the communion of the saints, which we affirm, but which we often do not feel. Help us be faithful for those who follow us, building courage into them rather than adding to their uncertainty.

May we be unusually aware of your presence today.

Amen.

1. "For All the Saints", text by William Walsham How. In the public domain.

A prayer for the thirty-second Sunday in Ordinary Time

God.

Half my friends are mad at half my friends who are mad at them.
And you and I both know that mad isn't the right word. But frustrated.
And concerned and critical and annoyed.

They have been getting that way for months.
They've been listening to news reports and opinions. They've been reducing each other to elevator pitches, one sentence that sums up everything sufficiently to abandon relationships. And respect. And love which you said even extends to our enemies.

And I haven't been able to help them, because I've been watching half my friends walking through the valley of the shadow of death.

God, we need you.

We need your help to remember to yield our hearts to you. We need your help to remember that your control of all things includes our involvement in the work you have called us to, and that work includes loving enemies and caring for widows and orphans and forgiving our brother and sister over and over again, and comforting those who mourn and choosing to serve you more than serving idols.

Help us see our idols.
Help us serve you.
We ask in the name of the one who served us to the death and back.

Amen.

+++

Reflecting on Joshua 24

A prayer for the thirty-third Sunday in Ordinary Time

God.

It seems like your people are always in trouble.
Sometimes it's because we get in trouble.
Sometimes it's because troubled times get us.

We are always looking for a leader to get us out of trouble, so we can go back to normal because we want to be safe. And have peace. Someone like Deborah.
But if we're honest with ourselves and you, we confess, sometimes we are in trouble because we don't confess.
The reason Deborah was an amazing judge, the reason she called out Barak's leadership and Sisera's demise, and Israel's deliverance was that you spoke to her. And you spoke to her because Israel cried out to you. And Israel cried out to you because they had rebelled against you and you let them suffer the consequences of their choices.

God, give us the discernment to stay out of the trouble we get in.
Give us the courage to choose to stay awake.
Give us the willingness to put on faith and hope and love, as if we are putting on clothing, as if we are staying awake, as if we are getting ready to see you soon.

And then when there is trouble, we can meet it with gracious dependence on you rather than fear of you.

We ask this through Christ our Lord.
I mean you.

Amen.

+++

Reflecting on Judges 4:1-10 and 1 Thessalonians 5:1-11

131

A prayer for the Feast of the Reign of Christ

God.

It's hard to talk about your kingdom and you being a king.

We pray all the time that your kingdom will come on earth as it is in heaven. That your will will be done on earth as it is in heaven. But we don't trust leaders and we want our independence. And we don't like the pain and confusion we see and feel.

And I think part of our resistance to you is the pictures we have of you. Forgive us the pictures we've created of you.

We think you are chasing us like a wolf when you are seeking us like a shepherd. We are worried about what people think of us when you think of us constantly. We cannot understand what you are doing to us. Why you are doing this to us. What you are allowing to happen to us.

You are telling a story much richer than we can understand. To be honest, even if we understood it, I'm not sure we'd like it.

Paul asked that you would give people a glimpse of you, enough that even if they didn't always like what you did, they would begin to trust your love. I ask that, too.

Give us a glimpse of a king that is a servant, a shepherd, and a sovereign.
Help us see a king that is compassionate and capable.
Remind us of a king that is self-sacrificing and worthy of receiving honor.

Help us know you, Christ, our once and always and future king.

Amen.

+++
Reflecting on Ezekiel 34:11-16, 20-24 and Ephesians 1:15-23

A prayer for those still stuck in 2020 (6/25/2020)

God.

The easiest thing in the world is to get frustrated.

To get frustrated with ourselves
when we can't do what we think we know how to do.
To get frustrated with others
when they don't do what we think they should.
To get frustrated with you
when you don't fix what we think you should.

When we're stretched thin with fatigue and worry, it's harder to stay encouraged.

So today, I ask you to encourage our hearts.

Even when others seem to make our work harder, help us to understand their lives, to provide for their needs, to find satisfaction and even delight in our good work.

And in our frustration, speak your peace, I ask.

Through Christ our Lord.

Amen.

We're halfway through this year (6/30/2020)

God.

We're halfway through this year. We have lots of stories about 2020.
What more could happen? What will be the next thing?
We want to be hopeful.
Some of us anticipate the worst.
For some of us, it's our job. For some of us, it's our personality.

I ask that you will help us today to anticipate you.
To listen for your whispers of peace.
To look for your fingerprints in the opportunities around us.
To accept your words of comfort and encouragement.
To offer our hands as yours.
To know that your mercies are new each morning.

We ask through Christ our Lord.

Amen.

A prayer for the active observers (7/2/20)

God.

As chaplains, we remember to weep with those who weep.
But some of us are not as good at rejoicing with those who rejoice.
And each day with our coworkers, we see many opportunities to rejoice.

We watch people figure things out.
We watch people care for messy things.
We hear people find the right words.
We see people day after day, in simple ways, offer excellent care.

In the middle of difficulty, we can rejoice in good work, in diligent use of the skills and experience you have given.

Help us, God, to help each other see reasons to rejoice.
Even as we pray together right now.

Amen.

What one person caring for people in hospitals looks for (7/3/20)

I haven't written much about the pandemic. I've been too busy living in the middle of it, going to work as a hospital chaplain. We continued to work, though with constant adjustments in ways we provided care to patients, their families and friends, and our coworkers.

Now that I'm starting to recover my equilibrium, I want to mention the things that I pay attention to.

I am fundamentally interested in the person in front of me. Sick or injured, worried or grieving, exhausted or frustrated or angry or numb. As much as I can debate the numbers and the trends and the patterns, all of those are not the person in front of me.

I'm more interested in hospitalizations than cases. When cases increase, it can be due to more cases or more identified cases. While those are useful numbers for many people, I'm affected by increases in hospitalizations. Those numbers aren't due to testing, they are due to people being sick.

I'm interested in what are called "excess deaths." Every day, on average, in the United States, 7,700 people die. If we are seeing people die from a virus rather than other causes, that's one thing. If we are seeing people die from the usual causes and then an additional group from the virus, that's another thing. When I did some digging a month ago, in this country we had about 700 excess deaths a day. Which means that every day 700 more families than usual are dealing with the loss of a loved one.[1]

I'm curious about non-medical reasons for questioning guidelines, and

1. Editor's note: the statistics on 2020 deaths are not complete. At the time reflection was written, these excess death numbers were accurate based on reading at the time. However, we're unsure the source of those numbers at that time. Rather than eliminate the paragraph or attempt to reconstruct the numbers, we've chosen to leave it as is, reflecting the feelings at that moment.

how people who question guidelines about masks and other precautions are or are not people who question other guidelines. Because I care about the person in front of me, I wonder. And, because I care about the person in front of me, I wear a mask. It doesn't hurt me. It may help you.

I'm curious about the amount of passion about positions. I've often noticed that when tension suddenly goes up in a meeting, the reason for the emotional response is often not related to the topic, but to something deeper, more emotional.

I'm sensitive to the kinds of loss and accumulating grief that we have. There have been many losses: lives, jobs, insurance, security. The response to loss is grief. Recently, I talked with a person who spent their wedding anniversary in the hospital, facing complications from cancer treatment, learning of the death of a loved one in the pandemic. And the person said, "I should be more encouraging." I reviewed the reasons that the person was okay processing their grief.

I'm also aware that I have watched people who have a positive test for COVID-19 take their last breaths. And people with other illnesses or injuries take their last breaths. And all without families in the room. And none of them alone, but with nurses and patient care techs in the room, eyes filling with tears. And so I know that the illness is real, that the implications are widespread, and all death is painful.

I'm aware of the impact of word choices: Social distance rather than physical distance. Freedom of action rather than responsibility for each other. Back to normal in contrast to new normal in contrast to making wise choices. Flattening the curve as opposed to stopping the spread.

I'm not taking sides, arguing positions, or debating. Instead, I'm letting you know what I look for. Because, after all, you are in front of me, too.

A prayer when we are not enough (7/6/2020)

God.

Some days, we simply aren't sure.
We're not sure our contribution matters.
We're not sure our skills are enough.
We're not sure we'll have what we need for the conversations and the procedures and the challenges and the uncertainty in front of us.

But we are doing work that matters.
God, we have responsibility for the care of the people in front of us. And we have the opportunity to serve everyone they, and we, are connected to.

Give us wisdom that goes beyond our training.
Give us compassion that goes beyond emotions.
Give us courage that goes beyond bravado.
Give us peace that passes understanding.
Give us today what we need for today.
Bless the work of our heads and hands and hearts.

And at the end of whatever our day is, give us rest.

Amen.

I like Ruth, she said (7/17/2020)

She was in her hospital bed. I was looking through the window. And we were talking on the phone. That's what happens with precautions these days.

She wanted to have a visit from a chaplain. Her body isn't doing well and won't get better.

We talked for a bit. And then I asked her who her favorite Bible person was.

She thought for a bit, reviewed where she had learned stories, and then said, "Ruth. That's a person who always stood out as having a good story."

I agreed and reviewed a bit of her story. She was from another country, and followed her mother-in-law back to Israel. "She was an immigrant," I said. "And I'm guessing that she wasn't very well accepted."

I thought about the story, about Naomi feeling like an outcast, feeling bitter about life. I thought about Ruth, not sure how much language she knew. She ended up gleaning from the harvested field, picking up what grain hadn't been harvested by workers who had known famine in recent years. (That's why Naomi and her family had left in the first place, because of a famine.) Boaz's instructions to leave extra in the field and to have Ruth eat with his workers for her safety, suggest that the life of outsiders was dangerous in many ways.

"But Ruth was King David's great-grandmother," I said to the patient on the phone. "She was part of the story of Jesus."

"I always liked Ruth," she said. "I wouldn't have remembered all those things, but I knew she was special."

I prayed for her.

And I acknowledged to myself that I hadn't remembered those things until I talked about them, until I started conversing with the patient in the bed.

And that's why, after 3,000 posts, we're moving on to 3,001.[1] Because we need to keep thinking about the stories, remembering our favorites, listening for what we missed before.

And grateful that this woman, for some reason, found courage in Ruth's story.

1. This reflection was the 3,001 post at 300wordsaday.com. There had been a celebration about reaching 3,000 posts.

We are feeling fragile (7/21/20)

God.
We are feeling a little fragile, some of us,
from solving big problems,
from facing the same small challenge one hundred times in a row,
from wanting to rest from trying to focus and finding that it's harder than we thought,
from wanting to be normal and discovering that things never were.

Today may we find courage for the big problems, wisdom for the repeated small challenges, rest and focus and peace.
May we give up nostalgia and accept the next moment as a new opening for your power and our competency.

May we delight in serving people.
Like you did.

Amen.

On words and prayer and a hope for peace this weekend (7/24/2020)

"Words won't do anything."

I was reminded of that again this week while standing with a husband who was watching his wife in her last twenty hours of breathing. "Words won't do anything," he said.

He wasn't trying to get rid of me or shut me up. He was stating the fact that we both knew to be true. I stood with the family. He asked me to pray and I did. I went back the next day and watched her breathe. I went back awhile later and helped him grieve.

What was clear was that whatever words I had were not fixing anything. They were not changing anything. But they gave me an excuse to stay in his presence.

We didn't talk politics or policies or platitudes. I did pray, when he asked, for peace and for God's presence. And even those words didn't "do" anything, like a magic formula would do something. But acknowledging the moment and asking God to make her aware of his peace and presence seemed to do something.

+++

I am more aware than ever that words don't fix anything in those deep moments of loss AND that words used incautiously can do almost irreparable harm. James reminds us that the tongue can do great harm.

These days, the keyboard and touch screen are extensions of the tongue, of the voice. Things that once were confined to earshot now enter bloodshot eyes and exhausted hearts and destroy relationships.

May we have peace.

A prayer for those who can't work from home (8/20/20)

God.

We get to care for the people of a whole region.
Body, mind, spirit.

It's an awesome opportunity.
It's too great a responsibility for us to understand, most of us.

While we feel the burden for everyone and everything,
we can only help the person in front of us.
Clean the room in front of us.
Unravel the logistical logjam in front of us.
Discern the pain and confusion in front of us.

So I ask for wisdom that goes beyond our training.
Compassion that goes beyond emotion.
And acceptance that helping this person in front of me is how we care for the people of a whole region.

I ask this, God, for each of us today.

Amen.

Sometimes we are the last resort (8/21/20)

God.
Sometimes chaplains are the last resort.

When people, when communities, when coworkers have tried everything, they come to us. Like we come to you.
The obstacles people face seem, to them anyway, impossible.

And then we are there.
When people feel defeated, help us offer courage.

When people feel abandoned, help us offer compassion.

When people feel confused, help us offer clarity.

And when we are feeling those things, please give us your peace.

And give us each other.

Amen.

We are afraid we'll jinx things (8/24/20)

God.

We need calm.

We're almost afraid to say that word, or words like it. We are afraid we'll jinx things, that mentioning calm or quiet will cause chaos.

I think we may even be afraid to say "jinx" in a prayer.

But we need calm.
In our minds.
In our hearts.
In our souls.
In our actions.

I ask today, for my friends, that the voice that has said "fear not" will bring calming to our lives and allow us to bring calm to the chaos we face.

Thank you, God.
Amen.

Building tiny altars (8/28/20)

Triage is where people wait. Behind the double door is the Emergency Department, with rooms and monitors and staff and expertise and hope and answers. This side of the double door is uncertainty and pain and fear and chairs spread apart.

In the old days, there was a Bunn coffee maker, tended by the coworkers at the desk. Then there was a machine that made a cup at a time, outsourcing the production and decisions to the people with uncertainty and pain and fear.

And then everything changed. Visitors were gone, people sat in the chairs briefly, on their way back to the empty rooms and then up to the floor or out with provisional answers.

Eventually, visitors came back, one at a time, with green wrist bands. The coffee counter, however, stayed empty.

Until the other day. I walked through triage on my way to somewhere else. I looked at the coffee counter. And discovered that someone had built a tiny altar. Not to coffee. But to courage. There was one stone, cornflower blue, with neon green and orange lettering. "Be Brave."

When something significant happened in the Old Testament adventures with God, people would make a pile of stones. They served as acknowledgements that something significant had happened. They served as personal reminders for those involved that something happened. And they served as conversation starters for subsequent generations. "What do these stones mean to you," God said that future generations would say of the pile of stones at the edge of the Jordan.

I know nothing of the person who left this stone in triage. I don't know whether it's an acknowledgement, a reminder, or a conversation starter. I do know that when I walked past, I was encouraged.

Not just at the end (8/31/20)

I went to the hospital room to visit.

It was a relaxed visit on a calmer day than usual. Less frantic, less catastrophic. And in this room, the mood was less catastrophic. The patient was ready to leave.

He knew that the diagnosis was the drug itself. Change the medication and things will be fine. And so we were talking about life and death with a little less urgency than I often hear.

He was sitting on the built-in sofa next to his wife.

"It's not my time," he said, looking at me, the chaplain. "But when I know my time is getting near, I'll have some long conversations with God."

I smiled.

"You know," I said, "If you said that about her, she'd be pretty upset."

I looked at his wife.

He looked up.

"She'd love to have a relationship with you all along, not just at the end."

She smiled and looked at him.

They weren't newlyweds. Forty years or so of knowing each other. Nearly thirty years married. We'd talked enough to know that they had been through some difficult times and that they loved each other. The kind of love that expressed in an affectionate picking on each other, debating small points with each other, ignoring the smart-aleck comments and encouraging each other in the middle of worry.

The kind of interaction that has grown from daily interaction about deep and irrelevant stuff. The kind of interaction that doesn't happen in lives lived at a respectful distance from each other.

The kind of relationship that becomes the whole life, not the kind of relationship resurrected at the last minute.

I think he understood.

A prayer for the anxious (9/8/2020)

God.

We read the news.
It makes us anxious.

Anxious for our families, for our communities, for our world.

We wonder, sometimes worry, what will happen.

Will we be enough? Can we do enough?
Will the people who make decisions make the right ones?
Will those of us who make decisions, make the best one?

God.

You know the news, too.
It doesn't make you anxious at all.

You care about our families, our communities, our world.

You are enough.

Give us your peace and your presence and your wisdom.
Enough for today, at least.

Please. Thank you.

Amen.

We need the calm (10/28/20)

God.

One of the things Jesus is known for is bringing calm to stormy seas.

In fact, one of the disciples, John or Peter or maybe Nathaniel one day asked, "Who is this that the wind and the waves obey him?"

We've got the storms right now.
We need the calm.

So for each of us, for the particular storm we are in, the one we are fighting, we are facing, would you please speak peace in us and through us?

Amen

Excess grief (10/31/20)

Dear friends.

Some of you know that I see people who die, sometimes before, sometimes after. It's what chaplains do at our hospital. In that process, I see diagnoses, I see cause of death. Sometimes it's related to COVID-19. Sometimes it isn't.

This isn't about that debate.

I keep talking to friends who are sad. They wonder whether there is always this sadness or if this year is different somehow. It is different somehow. In many ways.

This isn't about all of those ways.

This is about excess death.

In the United States, from January 26 through October 3, 299,000 more people died than would have been expected to die based on the number of deaths during the previous five years. Said differently, people die all the time from all causes. This year, about 300,000 more people than usual have died.

Of course, when you read the report in order to debate with me, you'll see that there are qualifiers about reporting lag (so the number is on the low side) and some averaging by week. I would love for you to read the report that carefully.

But *regardless of the cause,* these people died. Moms and grandpas. Aunts and nephews. Best friends and mentors. Babies we never had a chance to meet and 91-year-olds. Human beings who have no known next of kin. *Regardless of cause,* for eight months, about 1,234 more per day died (on average) than the 7,778 people (on average) than usually die.

No wonder so many of us are sad and angry and frustrated and numb.

151

No wonder we are reacting more than responding, that we want to punch walls and people, that we are denying and rationalizing. No wonder we don't know what to say to each other.

Because our culture isn't great at talking about death. And we've got many more lost people to not talk about.

Tomorrow is All Saints' Day, a day in the life of the church where we can remember those who are gone and their connection to God and to those who are here. Charlotte Donlon writes about how the words and texts of that day can provide support these days.

In a few hours, I'll be leading a funeral for a family. There will be many other families facing those moments today, more than on average. And this weekend, and last week.

I have no political agenda in this, just a chaplain agenda.

The grief is piling up. This is hard.

A prayer for the end of Daylight Saving Time (11/2/20)

God.

We're tired today.

We were supposed to get an extra hour of sleep on Sunday, but what we got was disrupted.
Our sleep is off, daylight is off, we're a little off.
One more thing to adjust to in a year of adjustment.

So today, I don't have anything fancy or deep to ask for, God.
Just for rest and strength.

And a little patience with ourselves and each other.

Amen

An old prayer that still matters (9/25/2020)

God.

"Out of the depths we cry to you, O Lord."[1]

That's what an ancient pray-er said to you.

And I'm guessing that those words are heard in our rooms every day.

For the patient with a hard diagnosis.
For the code team who worked hard to save a life.
For the coworker carrying difficult news from home.

For our community. For our country.

"Out of the depths we cry to you."

But God, we cry to you because you know our depths,
Because you are present with us there and always,
Because you can give us comfort and wisdom and courage and peace.

So today, we cry out to you, with honest desperation and threadbare confidence that you are there to cry to. But we are grateful that your presence doesn't depend on our confidence but on your compassion.

Through Christ our Lord.

Amen.

1. Psalm 130:1

The end of the year

And then the liturgical year ended.

After Christ the King, we started a new year with Advent 2020. A month later, we started the new calendar year with 2021.

Many people talked as if the new year would bring the end to the virus, to the fear, to the systemic injustice. Turning the calendar page doesn't make anything go away. Pandemics and pain do not conform to our schedules.

That said, we benefit from acknowledging seasons and cycles. Other books can take up the new liturgical year, the next phase of the virus, the next set of prayers. This year is done.

There are some loose ends, however. It seemed appropriate to think about thanks at the end of the year. It seemed appropriate to talk honestly about how to think about holiday gatherings after this kind of year. It seemed appropriate to reflect on some of the language we used.
And I did get a shot.

A prayer with thanks at the end of the year

God.

We need to be honest.

It's hard to be grateful for all the loss and grief this year.
For some of us, this has been the hardest year we've ever seen.

Thank you that you don't expect us to be happily grateful for the loss of
loved ones.
And yet, thank you that you are with us in that loss.

And there are things that we are grateful for.
Thanks for the remarkable people we work with.
Thanks for all the days we weren't sure we would make it,
and we did.

Thanks for a thousand decisions we needed wisdom for,
and found it.
Thanks for thousands of acts and conversations through which
our patients,
our community,
our coworkers knew that we cared as we walked away.
Thanks for a thousand moments in which we had
the courage we needed,
the peace that we needed,
the rest that we needed.

When we had what we needed.

God,
Thank you for us.
Thank you for you.

Amen.

Grief and holidays in 2020 (11/7/2020)

We're exhausted, many of us. We can't quite figure out why. We can't think as clearly as usual, we don't have the motivation we used to. Our relationships are struggling, we're more cranky.

We think that there may be something wrong with us. But there isn't. It's grief. Grief is our response to loss. Our responses can be physical, emotional, mental, spiritual, or a mix of all of those. And we've had a lot of loss this year.

The next months are full of family gatherings, holidays, and the expectations and routines that go with those. We wanted to give you some things to tell yourself as you approach the end of this year, to help you through what may be difficult.

Acknowledge that the last year has been hard.
When we look at our lives and our losses, we often think, "But their life is harder" or "I should be able to handle this" or "I have to be strong for my family." This year, however, there have been many kinds of loss and they all add up. Lost jobs, lost vacations, lost classrooms, lost routine, and lost loved ones. All that loss adds up. So, looking in the mirror, looking at each other, and saying "This IS hard" gives us the freedom to start addressing the pain and the grief.

Give yourself and others permission to hurt.
We know that we do hurt because of the loss. But some of us don't like to admit that we are hurting. Covering it doesn't help it. Acknowledging that your family can be sad because you lost a grandparent is important.

Acknowledge that everyone is feeling the loss differently.
For some people, this was a close friend. For others, this was someone they hardly knew. Rather than expecting everyone to be experiencing grief the same way, identify how you feel and know that someone else may feel differently. And be courageous enough to talk about how hard it is to talk about things.

Embrace adjustments in the traditions.
Gatherings will be challenging enough this year. Families and friends will be considering whether it's safe to gather, whether it's safe to talk about all that's happened in the world this year. For you, however, everything is personal. Someone is missing. So, make sure you intentionally talk about the traditions linked to that person.

You may want to consider whether a particular role or task the person did can be passed on to someone else or should be retired. If dad always lit the first candle, then talk about passing that role to the firstborn. If mom always fixed a fruitcake but no one else liked fruitcake, it's okay to retire that tradition. Every family has traditions, and some can be retired. (And you may want to start a new tradition!)

Words matter (11/25/2020)

I am a words guy. And I'm getting worse.

My friends come to me for words sometimes. They are looking for the right word for a moment, for a situation. Sometimes, I confess, I inflict my struggle against imprecision on others.

I care about words because words evoke meanings in us. They trigger memories, they shape how we think about situations.

I've remained mostly silent about four words, but it's time to talk.

Social. Virtual. Alone. Nuance.

We've been talking about *social distancing*, which conveys something about a gap in relationship. It feels akin to emotional distancing. But we could have been talking about ***physical*** distance, the space between bodies. We know how to work with physical distance, we work with that all the time through text and phone and FaceTime and letter-writing. We have worked with long-distance relationships for generations. But as soon as we made it social, we created a different feeling. And we got defensive.

We've been talking about *virtual* activities, a word that was related to simulation and hypothetical and games. Virtual reality is made-up, or it was for a long time. We put virtual backgrounds in our Zoom calls to hide the real background. But we could have been talking about on-line activities or mediated activities. We talk about virtual meetings and forget that these are real meetings in which real humans make actual decisions about life-changing situations happening through a variety of communication tools. We talk about virtual memorial services and forget that we are real people remembering the real death of a real person.

We've been talking about people dying alone. Which, before the current pandemic, happened often at the hospital and elsewhere. But we could have been talking about people dying without their family in the room.

And at the same time being treasured by the people who were caring for them. I've watched as people have died, hand being held by a nurse. Who then, of course, walked out of the room in tears. That person wasn't alone.

We've not talked about nuance. We could have talked about where masks are helpful and where they don't matter. We could have talked about what gatherings are worst and why, and what gatherings are safest, and why. We could have been more clear. We could have been more thoughtful. We would have been more helpful.

Peace.

I hate shots, but I'm on the list (12/18/2020)

I hate shots. I can't watch other people get them. I turn my head all the time in the hospital when a needle shows up anywhere close to an arm. And choosing to receive flu shots has been a challenge, though I've done it.

So when I cried about scheduling a shot the other day, you might think that I was going back to my childhood fears.

I wasn't.

I had just spent some time in our hallways where the physical, emotional, and spiritual effects of COVID-19 are being experienced by people infected, by their families, and by my co-workers. I'd sat with a spouse for a long time who was trying to figure out personal responsibility for this impersonal virus. While I was talking with that spouse, my colleague and friend attended the death of a person I'd responded to earlier in the day. I'd walked by the room where my first COVID-19 death was, where I had watched a nurse using her own phone to Facetime with the family before we'd started to figure out how to do it with hospital tablets.

And now I walked into the office with my friend and we each had an email with a link that would allow us to receive the Pfizer COVID-19 vaccine.

I was a bit overwhelmed.

Nancy and I had talked earlier about what I would do if it were offered, whether or not I should accept. If she had questions, I wanted to take that into account. She didn't hesitate. "Yes," she said.

And so, when I got the email, I scheduled the shot. And teared up.

I let Nancy know. She said "Thank you." I texted our kids. They celebrated. And I understood that every time I walk into work, aware of the risks and the realities, they walk in, too.

Unlike them, I am always aware of those whose work is more hands-on. The respiratory therapists, the patient care techs, the nurses. They put on the hair coverings and the masks and the goggles and the gloves and the gowns, and walk into the rooms. They provide the actual touch, the unmediated voice, the eye contact.

I forget, in the comparisons, that we as chaplains are not in THOSE rooms, but we are in the space, too. And the families of all of us are there. So I'm getting the vaccination.

I almost didn't say anything in public about being on the list.

Among the people I know and love are people for whom this action is political. For whom it is spiritual weakness. Fortunately, a friend reminded me that my action and words may be helpful to someone else.

I understand that on Wednesday, after the shot, I may be in the tiny, tiny percentage of bad side effects. Chaplains think about those things because we spend time with the 1% of bad outcomes and the 100% death rate among humans. But I'm not so much afraid of the virus or the shot as I am acutely aware of the implications of both in lives, and given the choice, I'm getting the shot.

I'm grateful for the privilege for protection. And for the opportunity to go to work. And for the blessing to be part of the lives, and yes, the deaths, of people.

Peace.

This is it (12/31/20)

God.

This is it. The last prayer together this year.

We've talked to you a lot this year, here and in patients' rooms and at kitchen tables all across northeast Indiana.

We've been surprised at what we've survived.
We're weary with the grief we've shared.
We're amazed at the incredible work of our coworkers, and even, if we admit it, our own good work.

And so, God, as we are here now, thank you for your strength and peace.

Please give us some rest as we end the year.
And give us courage for the next.

Amen.

Afterword: Becoming a chaplain in a pandemic by Jana Vastbinder

December 2019, a couple weeks after Jon started writing the prayers in this book, I became a Parkview Hospital chaplain. In our department, we often say chaplaincy is a calling. That was definitely the case for me, as I never wanted to work in a hospital. Honestly, the thought of blood and needles makes me cringe. I had been building a counseling ministry at a local church for the last five years and was just about to pass my test to become a licensed mental health counselor. My job of overseeing care ministries at the church was literally designed for me, but through a series of events, conversations, and promptings, God showed me He had other plans for my future. In October I applied to be a chaplain and started referring to the transition as a "new adventure" that only God could be leading. I had no idea what an adventure my first year in chaplaincy would be.

I had been used to meeting with people to process their darkest moments in life as a counselor. When I became a chaplain, suddenly my job was to be with people during those dark moments. A chaplain's role is to step into the deaths, traumas, anxieties, and unknowns with patients, families, and staff to offer a calming and empathetic presence. We help people navigate a range of unknowns. In my first couple months, even those procedures that were known to other staff were still unknown to me. I went into almost every shift with some level of anxiety wondering what difficult situation I would encounter during my eight to twelve hours there.

At the end of February, 2020, I was finally feeling more comfortable. And when I say "comfortable," I mean I didn't start every shift with a pit in my stomach, fervently hoping and praying for no catastrophes to occur while I was there! I will never be able to account for all the unknowns one faces in the hospital, but I'd been around long enough that I had a sense of what I was doing and who I could go to when I had questions. At that time, I was able to tell my family and friends I enjoyed what I did with some semblance of confidence. The following month, that confidence wavered as the pandemic came to our hospital system.

The policies and procedures I had begun to grasp changed drastically. Instead of walking the newly familiar hallways and units, we started calling patient rooms from our office. I had learned the etiquette of comforting families in the lobby or consult room and escorting them to bedside. Now, I had to inform them of the current visitation policy and offer condolences from afar. The weight and reality of unknowns both intensified and multiplied. Not only was I unsure of how to conduct myself at work, but then I would go home and try to navigate how to interact with my family and the rest of the world. None of us knew what to do or how to handle all the changes. Or what to do with the fear and questions of whether I could bring the virus home with me.

During my first couple monthly staff meetings, we talked about activities our team could do to bond in 2020. We talked about baseball games, cookouts, competitions, and retreats. I was excited to get to know my new team outside of work. Everything changed, and we ended up bonding, but it was over navigating uncharted territory and checking in with one another on how we were processing these historical moments. Instead of weekend plans, vacations, family activities, or even the weather, my conversations with coworkers started to revolve around what the best sanitizing process was once we came home from our shifts and how we and people we loved were coping with the shattering of what we called normal. We also focused on how to care well for others around the hospital system, but in socially distanced ways. While I felt seen and cared for by my colleagues and leaders, I was entrenched again in unknowns. But now we were all trying to figure it out together.

One step my leaders took to care for us was to start a resource called The Daily Dose. These short, daily videos were designed to encourage and connect coworkers. Several people had started working from home and were craving community. Others of us were giving direct patient care and were struggling with exhaustion. Everyone was dealing with a variety of needs, questions, and changes. The videos included interviews with people from across the organization on how they were coping with the pandemic. Each video concluded with a prayer from a chaplain. The Daily Dose was a reminder that we weren't alone, and we had physical, emotional, and spiritual resources available to us.

I started praying on the Daily Dose at the start of April. After fighting through my discomfort with being filmed, as well as with the adjustment of writing down my prayers for others (yet another new experience for me), I started to witness benefits from the videos. First, I felt more connected to the purpose and people of Parkview. Being so new to the organization, I didn't know many of the leaders or other departments within the system. I also watched as those leaders sought to care for employees and were proactively attempting to meet needs and give answers in the ever-shifting climate around us. Parkview strives to help the patients who come our way, but we also realize that our coworkers are part of those patients, families, and communities we serve.

As a counselor, I'm familiar with the power that comes from putting words to experiences and becoming aware of thoughts and feelings. The Daily Dose put that power on display. Through prayer, and describing thoughts and feelings, I watched as my fellow chaplains brought words and meaning to people's experiences. Jon, in particular, became a scribe of what felt like a never-ending season. He and other chaplains attempted to capture the concerns and needs of the hundreds of people we interact with on a regular basis. They touched on fear, uncertainty, confusion, anger, anxiety, depression, loneliness, pain, exhaustion, and grief – feelings that were tangibly present, but don't always like to be named. Capturing what we experience can bring connection. That moment where you think, "Hey, me too! I can relate." Or, as I found myself thinking, "Oh, that's why I feel the way I do." Words brought comfort and reasons and space to what was happening in and around us. We needed connection in 2020. Connection to people and understanding and grace. Chaplains attempted to help people make those connections and point people to God. I was able to be both a facilitator and participant in that encouragement.

As I continued to wrestle with the unknowns, difficult experiences, and my "new adventure," I noticed an urgency to grow in my faith. I knew if I wasn't being filled spiritually, I'd have nothing to give to those around me. I was also confronted with my dependence on God. No one could offer, or help me accept, comfort and assurance like Him. After all, He was the one who had led me into chaplaincy right before a pandemic. I grew in confidence that God knew what He was doing when He called me there. I was also dependent on my coworkers and community to try to make sense of what I had stepped into as a new chaplain. In the midst of all the changes, I made a goal for myself: to be faithful with what God put in front of me. To do as best as I could, giving and accepting grace along the way, and taking it one step at a time. One situation at a time. One person at a time. Sometimes that person was me. And often, I needed to start with prayer. And when I didn't have the words, I relied on the prayers of those around me. Prayers like those found in this book.

Jana Vastbinder is a hospital chaplain. Previously, she was a care ministry director and counseling coordinator in a church, and is a licensed mental health counselor. Jon and Hope met Jana when the girls were stuck watching their brothers play soccer in middle school.

Resources on Faith, Sickness, Grief, and Doubt

In 2017, Patrick Riecke started working on his second book, about talking with sick, dying, and grieving people.[1] It was clear to him that this wasn't going to be one book about faith and doubt, sickness and grief. His experience as a pastor and chaplain and leader and grieving father told him that this needed to be the first in a series of resources.

There are five books in the series. Each book is practical and honest, with explanations and resources based in personal and professional experience. To find out the latest additions to this series, visit EmeraldHopePublishing.com

Patrick Riecke, *How to Talk With Sick, Dying, and Grieving People: When There Are No Magic Words to Say*. (Fort Wayne, Emerald Hope Publishing House, 2018).

Patrick Riecke, *How to Find Meaning in Your Life Before it Ends*. (Fort Wayne, Emerald Hope Publishing House, 2019).

Jon Swanson, *Giving a Life Meaning: How to Lead Funerals, Memorial Services, and Celebrations of Life*. (Fort Wayne, Emerald Hope Publishing House, 2020).

Kristen and Patrick Riecke. *No Matter How Small: Understanding Miscarriage and Stillbirth*. (Fort Wayne, Emerald Hope Publishing House, 2020).

Jon Swanson, *"God. We Need You": A Year of Prayer in a Hospital Chapel*. (Fort Wayne, Emerald Hope Publishing House, 2020).

---

1. His first book was his master's degree thesis. He published it as an experiment in publishing.

About the author

Rev. Dr. Jon Swanson spent 2020 working as a hospital chaplain three days a week. Living through his own challenges led to this book.

It builds on many threads. He's an ordained pastor with 15 years in church ministry. He's spent more than 20 years in higher education, teaching communication, management, and spiritual formation, and working as an administrator. Most recently, he's worked as a hospital chaplain in a Level II Trauma Center, an adjunct professor, and a consultant with churches and non-profits. And he's written about grief, prayer, Advent, Lent, and spiritual journeys.

Nancy and Jon have been married since 1983 and have two married children and a daughter in heaven. They've walked regularly since 2006, and he started running in 2014.

If this book – or any of Jon's books – have been helpful, please leave a review on Amazon.

Books (all available at anewroutine.com)

Anticipation: An Advent Reader (2012)

Learning A New Routine. Reading the Sermon on the Mount a Little Bit at a Time (2012)

Lent for Non-Lent People: 33 Things to Give up for Lent and Other Readings (2013)

A Great Work: A Conversation With Nehemiah For People (Who Want To Be) Doing Great Works (2013)

Saint John of the Mall: Reflections for the Advent Season (2017)

Giving a Life Meaning: How to Lead Funerals, Memorial Services, and Celebrations of Life. (2020)

"God. We Need You": A Year of Prayer in a Hospital Chapel. (2020)

Before You Walk In: A Devotional Primer for Chaplains and Pastoral Visitors (2020) at beforeyouwalkin.com.

Giving A Year Meaning: A Healing Journal for Advent 2020 (2020)

Blogs

300wordsaday.com – I write six days a week about following God. Each Sunday is a prayer.

socialmediachaplain.com – I write regularly about caring for others, particularly in hospitals.